DEVELOPMENT NGOs FACING THE 21ST CENTURY

Perspectives from South Asia

Edited by:
JUHA VARTOLA
MARKO ULVILA
FARHAD HOSSAIN
TEK NATH DHAKAL

Institute for Human Development
Kathmandu 2000

Published by:
Institute of Human Development
Lekhnath Marg, Thamel - 29,
Kathmandu, Nepal
Tel: +977 1 414623
E-mail: drtika@col.com.np

In association with:
Coalition for Environment and Development, Finland and
Vasudhaiva Kutumbkam – Lokayan (Global Responsibility Forum), India

Price: NPR 400

Printed by: Sewa Printing Press
Kathmandu, Nepal

ISBN 99933-310-0-6

CONTENTS

PREFACE

Factors leading to 'market failures' and 'government failures' coupled with an alternative mechanism which may have a 'comparative advantage' has engendered the emergence of non-governmental organisations (NGOs) since the early of 1970s. NGOs are believed to have a mechanism of addressing the needs of majority of the people. They can do so by aggregating public goods, conserving environment, creating safety nets for the powerless and helping diverse sections of the populace to promote development. This sector has also been taken presumed as one the key actors of today's development discourse for the socio-economic development of the people at the grassroots level. NGOs particularly in developing countries are assuming various roles ranging from relief, advocacy, education and social movements to empowerment of downtrodden and deprived section of the society. In multicultural communities, the pluralist sense of social justice has become the overriding concern of both Northern and Southern NGOs. However, NGOs are not the substitutes of the State, for their success lies more in building and strengthening indigenous social, cultural and ecological institutions and connecting them to universal knowledge and acting as praxis for fostering long-term national, regional and global development process.

Looking into the growing number of NGO, diversified functional areas and their causes and consequences, which might have significant impacts upon the national politics and local lives, the functioning of NGOs has become an area of interest from different perspectives. There exist, however, misconceptions in different quarters including among NGOs themselves about NGO roles and effectiveness and sustainability of their program activities. How to face this challenge and make this third sector more meaningful to fight poverty, illiteracy, poor health at a global scale globe has been a crucial issue in the 21st century. It could be helpful to wipe out such problems by dissemination of information their significant roles and activities and by way of knowing the NGOs more intimately. Unfortunately, literature available in the subject area is meagre. The present publication *'Development NGOs Facing the 21st Century: Perspectives from South Asia'* is an attempt to help the readers to understand more about NGOs and their roles in development and also to share the reality among the readers about some of the pertinent queries.

Institute for Human Development (IHD) is happy to bring this publication out amidst the readers. The opinions and ideas expressed in the articles are those of the authors. In fact, this publication is an outcome of the co-operation and financial support extended by Coalition for Environment and Development (CED), Finland. The editors of this book - Professor Juha Vartola of the University of Tampere and Researchers Marko Ulvila & Farhad Hossain of the

University of Tampere and Nath Dhakal - a research fellow of Tribhuvan University - have contributed a lot for conceptualising, organising and managing this project. In this context we would like to express our gratitude to all editors and co-partners for bringing this book out.

We hope the publication will be a useful document in satisfying the readers who are interested in the multifaceted development activities being carried out by the of NGOs. If this goal is achieved, then we feel ourselves encouraged, obliged and rewarded for bringing out this publication.

Krishna Devkota
Executive Member
Institute for Human Development (IHD), Nepal

FOREWORD

This book has benefited from two different kind of partnerships between South-Asians and Finns. The older one is the link between Indian and Finnish social movement activists, namely leaders from Lokayan in New Delhi and Service Centre for Development Co-operation and Coalition for Environment and Development (CED) in Finland. Since 1989 there has been intense dialogue between people associated with these organisations on number of issues. One of the central one has been the role of foreign funding in international solidarity, and more specifically on its impacts on the popular organisations and social movements.

One such dialogue 'Voluntarism in Nepal: Experiences and Reflection' was held on 4-5 April 1999 and co-organised by Centre for Study of Developing Societies (CSDS), New Delhi and Coalition for Environment and Development. It was part of a wider programme conducted by CSDS and sponsored by the Service Centre for Development Cooperation of Finland on democratising the north-south partnership in voluntary sector. The articles by Dr. Diwakar Chand, Dr. Krishna Bhattachan, Mr Dipak Gyawali and Mr. Gopal Siwakoti 'Chintan' originate from that meeting.

The other process from which this book stems is a joint research project 'NGOs in Development' that draws together scholars and post-graduate students from departments of public administration of the Universities of Dhaka in Bangladesh, Tampere in Finland and Tribhuvan University in Nepal. The project is lead by Prof. Juha Vartola at the University of Tampere and funded by the Academy of Finland. All the four editors and seven of the contributors of the book are engaged in this research project. Contributions by them and others from the research community provide new empirical findings to the work of NGOs from field and policy level.

These two processes - dialogue among social activists and joint research project by academic practitioners - were brought together in this book for cross fertilisation of ideas and bringing the too often separate realms of knowledge inside the covers of a one book. The present compartmentalisation of activities has lead to a situation where the academic community discusses mainly with each other in international journals and exclusive books. Similarly, the debate among social movements and non-governmental organisations is generally confined to their own meetings and publications. The separateness of the discussion hinders learning from the people in the other camps, and therefore impedes generation of knowledge that is based on both real life experiences and on academic inquiry. Therefore it was felt necessary to bring out a volume combing the two perspectives.

Coalition for Environment and Development and Vasudhaiva Kutmbkam - Lokayan are happy to act as co-publishers of this important volume. Through this cooperation the experiences from Nepal and elsewhere can be distributed more widely in South Asia and Europe.

Marko Ulvila
Chairman
Coalition for Environment and
Development, Finland

Vijay Pratap
Convenor
Lokayan - Vasudhaiva
Kutumbkam, India

Mr. Mokbul Morshed Ahmad is an Assistant Professor at the Department of Geography and Environment, University of Dhaka in Bangladesh. Currently he is a Doctoral Candidate at the Department of Geography, University of Durham, UK. His current research includes status of NGOs, their Field Workers, and Microcredit Finance in development management in Bangladesh.

Contact information: E-mail: dgg3mma@hotmail.com

Dr. Salahuddin Aminuzzaman is a Professor of Public Administration, University of Dhaka, Bangladesh. He is also the Director of the Center for Administrative and Development Studies (CADS), an independent research and consulting body. His area of specialisation includes: development management, policy analysis, programme/project management and institutional analysis. He has taught in University of Dar es Salaam, Tanzania; Seychelles Institute of Management, Seychelles; and North Dakota State University, USA. He has also wide experience as a consultant to selected UN agencies and international and national NGOs.

Contact information: Department of Public Administration, University of Dhaka, Dhaka-1000, Bangladesh. Tel.: +880 2 834495. Fax: +880 2 865583. E-mail: suddin@bangla.net

Dr. Afroza Begum is an Assistant Professor, Department of Public Administration, University of Chittagong, Bangladesh. Recently she has completed her Ph.D. degree in Public Administration. The topic of her doctoral dissertation was *"Government-NGO Collaboration in Development Management in Bangladesh: An Institutional Analysis"*. Her research interest includes local and urban government in Bangladesh and the role of NGOs in development. A book by her titled 'Government-NGO Interface in Development Management: Experiences of selected collaboration models in Bangladesh' is underway.

Contact information: Department of Public Administration, University of Chittagong, Chittagong, Bangladesh, E-mail: afroza@ctgu.edu

Dr. Krishna B. Bhattachan is one of the founding faculty members of the Central Department of Sociology & Anthropology of Tribhuvan University in Nepal. He is a Lecturer and former Head of the Central Department of Sociology at Tribhuvan University. Dr. Bhattachan received his Ph.D. at the University of California, Berkeley, USA in 1993. His areas of specialisation are development, ethnic and gender studies. He is one of the Nepal's most prolific writers in academic and popular media on the issues of development and ethnicity. He has published numerous articles in national & international books, journals, magazines and newspapers. Recently Dr. Bhattachan has edited a book *'Developmental Practices in Nepal'* jointly with Dr. Chaitanya Mishra.

Contact information: G.P.O. Box: 5353, Kathmandu, Nepal. Tel.: +977 1 528549 & +977 1 331852 Fax: +977 1 528049 E-mail: bhattachan@unlimit.com.

Dr. Diwakar Chand is a former Member-Secretary of the then Social Service National Co-ordination Council (SSNCC). He has been associated with Association of Development Agencies (ADAN) as a President since 1993, Currently, he is working as an Advisor of South Asian Fund Raising Group (with its regional office in New Delhi) and also working as the President of Nepal Fund Raising Group. He has authored over 7 books and numerous research article which has been published in national and international journals as well. He has received several awards and has also been decorated with Gorkha Dakshin Bahu from His Majesty the King.

Contact information: P.O. Box: 3184, Kathmandu, Nepal. Tel.: +977 1 271933 Fax: +977 1 434809 E-mail: chanda@mos.com.np

Mr. Gopal Siwakoti 'Chintan' is a Lecturer at the Faculty of Law, Tribhuvan University, and St. Xavier's College in Kathmandu. He is the founding Executive Director of Kathmandu-based International Institute for Human Rights, Environment and Development (INHURED International) and a General-Secretary of Rastriya Sarokar Samaj (National Concerns Society) which is a national network of local movements and activists. He has written widely on global environment, development and human rights issues. He holds Diploma Degree in Human Rights from the International Institute of Human Rights, Strasbourg, France, and LL.M. from the Washington College of Law, American University, Washington, DC.

Contact information: P.O.Box 2125, Kathmandu, Nepal. Tel: +977-1-429741 E-mail: inhured@mos.com.np

Dr. Govind P. Dhakal is the Head of the Central Department of Public Administration of Tribhuvan University in Nepal. His research interests are development administration, urban studies, and aid management in Nepal. He is the Executive Editor of the Public Administration Journal (PAJ) and the Public Administration Association of Nepal (PAAN) Journal.

Contact information: Central Department of Public Administration, Tribhuvan University, P.O.Box 1509, Kathmandu, Nepal. E-mail: cdpa@infoclub.com.np

Mr. Tek Nath Dhakal is a Lecturer of the Central Department of Public Administration of Tribhuvan University in Nepal. Currently he is a Doctoral Candidate of the Department of Administrative Science of the University of Tampere, Finland and working in the research project 'NGOs in Development', funded by the Academy of Finland. His current research work is on the role of NGOs in the development process of Nepal.

Contact information: Central Department of Public Administration, Tribhuvan University, P.O.Box 1509, Kathmandu, Nepal. E-mail: dhakaltn@ccsl.com.np

Mr. Dipak Gyawali is a member of Royal Nepal Academy of Science and Technology (RONAST). He is also associated with Interdiciplinary Analysts and Nepal Water Conservation Foundation.

Contact information: P.O. Box 3971, Kathmandu, Nepal, E-mail: ida@mos.com.np

Mr. Farhad Hossain is a Research Fellow at the Department of Administrative Science, University of Tampere, Finland. In the 1980s he was an NGO activist in Bangladesh. At present he is working in the research project 'NGOs in Development', funded by the Academy of Finland. His current research includes issues related to 'sustainability' and 'management capacity' of Nordic NGO-led development projects in Bangladesh and Nepal. He is teaching Intercultural Communication and Development Studies with main focus on NGOs. Recently Mr. Hossain has co-edited a book '*Learning NGOs and the Dynamics of Development Partnership*' jointly with Mr. Marko Ulvila and Ms. Ware Newaz.

Contact information: University of Tampere, Department of Administrative Science, FIN-33014 University of Tampere, Finland. Tel.: +358 50 3385833. Fax: +358 3 215 6020. E-mail: kumoho@uta.fi

Mr. F.R.M. Mortuza Huq is a practicing health official and a researcher from Bangladesh, currently working in health management information systems for the Wesley Hospital, Brisbane, Australia. He has worked with United Nations Development Programme (UNDP) and German Agency for Technical Cooperation (GTZ). He has an MBA degree in marketing and finance as well as a Masters in Public Administration. Currently he is pursuing a Masters Degree in Public Health (MPH) from the University of Queensland, Australia.

Contact information: suddin@bangla.net

M. Miles lives in Birmingham and studies the histories of social and educational responses to disabilities in Asia, the Middle East and Africa.

Contact information: 4 Princethorpe Rd., Birmingham B 29 5PX, UK. Tel/Fax: 44 121 472 4348, E-mail: m99miles@hotmail.com

Ms. Mari Poikolainen is a Research Fellow at the University of Tampere with the 'NGOs in Development' research project, funded by the Academy of Finland. She is an Anthropologist and also the Doctoral Candidate of the Department of Ethnology, University of Jyväskylä, Finland. Her research includes issues related to ethnicity, culture, NGOs and volunteers in Nepal and Finland.

Contact information: Department of Administrative Science, University of Tampere, FIN-33014 University of Tampere, Finland. Tel.: +358 3 215 7390 E-mail: makapo@cc.jyu.fi

Dr. Tika Prasad Pokharel is the Member-Secretary of the Social Welfare Council of His Majesty's Government of Nepal. He is also a Visiting Faculty of the Central Department of Public Administration of Tribhuvan University in Nepal and a senior scholar in the research project 'NGOs in Development', funded by the Academy of Finland. Dr. Pokharel has a wide practical and academic experience in development economics and NGO functioning in Nepal.
Contact information: P.O. Box 2948, Kathmandu, Nepal, E-mail: drtika@col.com.np

Mr. Mojibur Rahman is a Doctoral Candidate of the Department of Political Science, University of Helsinki, Finland. His current research includes issues related to poverty, child labour, child rights in Bangladesh and Nepal. Recently he has been working as a Research Fellow in the Nordic Institute of Asian Studies in Copenhagen, Denmark.
Contact information: rahman@sato.helsinki.fi

Ms. Shanti Bajracharya Rajbhandari is a Lecturer in Economics of the Padma Kanya (Girls) Campus of Tribhuvan University in Nepal. She is a Doctoral Candidate of the Department of Administrative Science of the University of Tampere, Finland and working in the research project 'NGOs in Development', funded by the Academy of Finland. Her research interests include issues related to gender, NGOs, and development in Nepal.
Contact information: GPO Box 7813, Kathmandu, Nepal. Tel: +977-1-535962 E-mail: green@kishor.wlink.com.np

Mr. A.K.M. Saifullah is a Doctoral Candidate of the Department of Administrative Science of the University of Tampere, Finland and working in the research project 'NGOs in Development' in Bangladesh, funded by the Academy of Finland. Recently he has completed his M.Phil. degree in Public Administration from the University of Dhaka, Bangladesh. His current research work is on the impact and relevance of NGO activities in the development management in Bangladesh.
Contact information: 260/1 East Goran, road No8, Dhaka 1219, Bangladesh. E-mail: rri@citechco.net

Mr. Marko Ulvila is a Research Fellow at the University of Tampere with the 'NGOs in Development' research project, funded by the Academy of Finland. He is studying the institutional landscape of Finnish NGO projects and partnerships in Bangladesh and Nepal. Mr. Ulvila is also active in Finnish citizens' organisations such as Friends of the Earth Finland and Coalition for Environment and Development.

Contact information: Department of Administrative Science, University of Tampere, 33014 University of Tampere, Finland. E-mail: marko.ulvila@uta.fi

Dr. Juha Vartola is a Professor of Public Administration at the Department of Administrative Science of the University of Tampere in Finland. He has more than 25 years of teaching and research experience in Public Administration. His areas of specialisation are organisation theory, administrative reform, security administration, European Union policy, and administrative science theories applied in developed and developing countries. He is the Director of the research project 'NGOs in Development', funded by the Academy of Finland.

Contact information: University of Tampere, Department of Administrative Science, FIN-33014 University of Tampere, Finland. Tel.: +358 3 215 6357 Fax: +358 3 215 6020. E-mail: hljuva@uta.fi

ACRONYMS AND ABBREVIATIONS

ABC Nepal:	A development NGO in Nepal
ADAB	Association of Development Agencies in Bangladesh
ADB	Asian Development Bank
ADP	Annual Development Programme
AGM	Annual General Meeting
AIDS	Acquired Immune Deficiency Syndrome
ASA	Association for Social Advancement
BASE	Backward Society Education
BASF	Bangladesh Shishu Adhikar Forum (Forum for Child Rights)
BBS	Bangladesh Bureau of Statistics
BGMEA	Bangladesh Garments Manufacturers & Exporting Association
BITI	BRAC Information Technology Institute
BONGOS	Business Organised NGOs
BRAC	Bangladesh Rural Advancement Committee
BRAVE	Bhutanese Refugee Aiding the Victim of Violence
BRDB	Bangladesh Rural Development Board
CARE	Committee for Assistance and Relief Everywhere
CARITAS	A Christian religious NGO
CBO	Community Based Organisations
CDO	Chief District Office/r
CHILD	Child Health Initiative for Lasting Development
CIDA	Canadian International Development Agency
CPN-UML	Communist Party of Nepal – United Marxist-Leninist
CRC	(UN) Convention on the Rights of the Child
CWIN	Child Workers In Nepal
DAC	Development Assistance Committee
DDC	District Development Committee
DONGOs	Donor Organised Non-Governmental Organisations
EPI	Expanded Programme on Immunisation
ERD	External Resource Division
FAMH	Frontier Association for the Mentally Handicapped
FD	Foreign Donation
FECOFUN	Federation of Community Forest Users, Nepal
FP-FP	Family Planning Facilitation Project
FUG	Forest Users Group
FY	Fiscal Year
GB	Grameen Bank (Rural Bank)

GDP	Gross Domestic Product
GK	Gonosastha Kendra (A Bangladeshi NGO in health sector)
GLA	Government Line Agencies
GNP	Gross National Product
GOB	Government of Bangladesh
GONGOs	Government Organised Non-Governmental Organisations
Gos	Governmental Organisations
GROs	Grassroots Organisations
GSS	Gono Sahajja Sangstha (A Bangladeshi NGO)
GTZ	Deutsche Gesellschaft fur Technische Zusammenarbeit (German Technical Assistance)
HDFC	Housing Development Finance Corporation
HPD	Health & Population Division
IFC	International Finance Corporation
IFS	Institutional Financial Self-sufficiency
IGG	Income Generation Group
IIRR	The International Institute of Rural Reconstruction
ILO	International Labour Organisation
INDRASS	Institute for National Development Research & Social Service
INGO	International Non-Governmental Organisations
IPEC	International Programme for Elimination of Child Labour
IPU	Inter Parliamentary Union
IVO	International Voluntary Organisation
JICA	Japan International Cooperation Agency
LWS	Lutheran World Service
MCH-FP	Mother & Child Health and Family Planning
MCI	Micro Credit Institution
MFI	Microfinance Institutions
MHC	Mental Health Center
MOHFW	Ministry of Health & Family Welfare
MP	Member of Parliament
MR	Mental Retardation / Mentally Retarded
MRC	Multidisciplinary Resource Center
NAB	NGO Affairs Bureau
NDI	National Democratic Institute
NEFAS	Nepal Foundation for Advanced Studies
NFE	Non Formal Education
NFOWD	National Forum of Organisations Working with the

	Disabled
NFPE	Non Formal Primary Education
NGOs	Non-Governmental Organisations
NORAD	Norwegian Agency for Development Co-operation
NPR	Nepali Rupee (Currency)
NSI	National Security Intelligence
NWAB	National Women's Association of Bhutan
NYAB	National Youth Associates of Bhutan
ODA	Overseas Development Assistance
OECD	Organisation for Economic Co-operation and Development
OFMP	Operational Forest Management Plan
Pos	Partner Organisations
Pos	Programme Organisations
PRA	Participatory Rural Appraisal
Proshika	A NGO in Bangladesh
PVDOs	Private Voluntary Development Organisations
PVOs	Private Voluntary Organisations
RDP	Rural Development Programme
Red Barnet	Save the Children-Denmark
Redd Barna	Save the Children-Norway
RSDC	Rural Self-reliance Development Center
RSPN	Royal Society for Protection of Nature
Rädda Barnen	Save the Children-Sweden
SCEMRB	Society for Care & Education of the Mentally Retarded, Bangladesh
SCF	Save the Children Fund
SCINOSA	Society for Children in Need of Special Attention
SDP	Self-reliance Development Programme
SFDP	Small Farmers Development Programme
SIP	Small Irrigation Projects
SSNCC	Social Service National Co-ordination Council
SWC	Social Welfare Council
Taka	Bangladeshi Currency (BDT)
Taksvärkki	Finnish Development NGO
TB	Tuberculosis
Thana	Sub-district in Bangladesh
UCEP	Underprivileged Children's Education Programme
UK	United Kingdom
UMN	United Mission to Nepal
UN	United Nations
UNDP	United Nations Development Programme

UNESCO	United Nations Educational Scientific and Cultural Organisation
UNHCR	United Nations High Commissioner for Refugees
UNICEF	United Nations Children's Fund
UPE	Universal Primary Education
US	United States
USA	United States of America
USAID	US Agency for International Development
USD	US$ / US Dollar
USE	Unitarian Service Committee
WAC	Women Awareness Center
WB	World Bank
VDC	Village Development Committee
WFP	World Food Programme
WHO	World Health Organisation
VHSS	Voluntary Health Services Society
Vos	Village Organisations
Vos	Voluntary Organisations
WTO	World Trade Organisation

PART 1 HIGHLIGHTING THE CONCEPTS AND ISSUES

1. INTRODUCTION: DEVELOPMENT NGOS FACING THE 21ST CENTURY

Juha Vartola

The role of Non-Governmental Organisations (NGOs) in has at the same time increased and changed its many faces in developing countries since the 1970s. OECD countries are putting more emphasis on NGOs as an alternative channel to transfer assistance to developing countries. National public administrations in Western countries are being downsized, and the same seems to happen in many developing countries, following the model of donor countries.. NGOs seem to be today one response to this need. Thus all kind of voluntary organisations are strategically more and more important for the future of the so called welfare states. On the other hand, NGOs have proved - at least to some extend - their effectiveness in managing development aid. Nevertheless still too little of their activities is known. The most important thing that we do not know is, what is the effectiveness - or as NGO jargon says, 'sustainability' of their functioning.

In order to overcome the global development challenges, i.e. fighting poverty, environmental degradation, and upholding human rights, equality and democracy in societies, serious NGOs need to find their way ahead. It must be remembered, unfortunately, that a growing part of 'angels of mercy'[1] are nothing but profit-making organisations. Practically, over the decades the size of the NGO field has increased and it has become more complex, much more quickly than the 'donor organisations' have been able to understand. This development scenario has received some attention from researchers. But the whole issue has mainly found publicity from evaluators and consultants hired by donor agencies or by the NGOs themselves. Thus, the initiative to generate well-founded knowledge about NGOs in development needs continuing evaluation also from the side of academic researchers in all social sciences. The factors which determine the success of their activities, their role and planned & non-planned effects in the local cultures where they operate, their organisation and management, their efficiency and effectiveness from the point of view of sustainability, are all questions that need more and more in-depth scientific work and co-operation from all academic social sciences.

Despite the recent economic advances in many parts of Asia, South Asia has remained backward in this respect. South Asia covers an small area of the total land mass in the world. However, some 1,13 billion people live there -

---

[1] Expression is from Tvedt 1998, *Angels of Mercy or Development Diplomats: NGOs and Foreign Aid.* London: James Currey.

roughly one fifth of the human race. During the eighties, the population growth rate in South Asia was 2.4 per cent as against 0.8 per cent for the developed world. Among the one billion poorest people in the world, 35 per cent lives in South Asia -- in terms of 'quality of life' South Asia's performance has remained generally poor. State failure and market failure are assumed to be responsible for this backward situation of the region. Since the 1970s, due to the poor performance of public and private agencies in development management, the donors have increasingly been involving NGOs in development management. However, the gap between the rich and the poor remained more or less unchanged throughout South Asia. Despite their comparative advantages in many sectors of development, present days the efficiency and effectiveness of NGOs are also being questioned. Therefore, academic understanding on the region and the existing development scenario is important. In this book we try to give some contributions to these complicated questions.

CONTENTS OF THE BOOK:

In general, the book discusses the comparative advantage and disadvantages of NGOs in the development process of South Asia, with a specific focus in Nepal. Findings of our recent research works in the region is also reflected in the book. This book is a combined effort of the authors, both from Finland and South Asia, and hence contains a significant outlook.

The book is divided into three parts. The first part discusses the concepts and issues. The second part is concentrated o the NGO activities in Nepal. The final part is discussing the NGO experiences from other South Asian countries.

Part I: Highlighting the concepts and issues

Marko Ulvila in his article introduces four different approaches to development NGOs. He calls them aid project management, neo-liberal advocacy, leftist critique and radical objection. With the examples from recent literature he attempts to bring some clarity into the very diverse NGO literature.

Farhad Hossain discusses the issue of project sustainability of NGO-led development initiatives. He presents the South Asian development scenario and analyses the sustainability of NGO initiatives in Bangladesh and Nepal. He analyses the issues and aspects of sustainability by highlighting the role of the donor, the recipient country, and the operating NGOs.

Mari Poikolainen focuses at cultural encounters in NGO settings of Finnish expatriates (volunteers and missionaries) in Nepal. She analyses interview material on the encounters utilising the concept of field. She argues that by dismantling the homogenising notions of the field it is possible to get a more diversified picture of NGOs.

Part II: NGO activities in Nepal

4

The second part is designed with the papers prepared by the scholars in Nepal. In his paper *Tika Prasad Pokharel* discusses the definitions of NGOs and present overall experiences of the NGO activities in Nepal. Furthermore, he highlights future challenges to NGOs and to other relevant agents.

Diwakar Chand first outlines the history of voluntarism in Nepal, and reflects on the role of voluntarism in Nepal today. Based on his vast experience and research, Chand makes suggestions for improved policy environment and new perspectives for voluntary action in Nepal.

Krishna B. Bhattachan's paper discusses NGOs from the perspective of Nepal's diverse ethnic composition. He draws attention to indigenous forms of voluntarism and reflects on the ways international and local NGOs have dealt with the various nationalities of Nepal.

Tek Nath Dhakal writes about the policy perspective of NGO operation in Nepal in terms of their growing numbers, diversified functional areas, their causes and consequences, which might have significant impacts upon the national politics and local lives. He analyses the Eighth Plan 1992-1997 & Ninth Plan 1997-2002 and the measure taken by His Majesty's Government of Nepal in institutionalising the NGOs as a development partner of the country.

Dipak Gyawali presents the basic contradictions in the development discourse and practice, and assesses the place of NGOs in the structures. He notes that in Nepal the state-market-civil society formation is far from ideal, and this can be attributed to both indigenous and exogenous factors. Drawing from an example of one of the older Nepali NGOs, Swabalamban, he discusses the controversial role of donor agencies.

In his chapter *Govind P. Dhakal* locate NGOs as part of the autonomous civil society in Nepal. He highlights the importance of good governance, democracy and institutional pluralism in strengthening the civil society. The challenges of Nepali society in achieving these positive elements and the potential role of NGOs are addressed in the paper.

Shanti Bajracharya Rajbhandari discusses the problem of girl trafficking and the responses by the NGOs to the pressing concern. As examples, she present three leading Nepali NGOs in the field and assesses their activities in the issue.

Gopal Siwakoti 'Chintan' presents a case of foreign intervention in Nepal's left politics. He outlines the fragmentation and transformation of the left after the restoration of democracy and describes the role foreign funding and NGOs in it.

Part III: Experiences from South Asia

In the final part of the book *M. Miles* in his chapter reviews contrasting patterns of 'Disability NGO' development in Pakistan and Bangladesh. After sketching the historical background, the focus of his paper is on mental retardation (MR) service organisations from the early 1980s to mid 1990s, a period during which those NGOs expanded, mostly with foreign assistance.

Mokbul Morshed Ahmad presents an outline of the overall situation of NGOs in Bangladesh, then set out the legal issues in detail and finally make proposals for improvements. Laws i.e. acts, ordinances, regulations, circulars, etc. practised by the NGO Affairs Bureau (NAB) of the Government in managing NGO activities has been presented in the chapter. His paper also presents an understanding on State-NGO relation in Bangladesh.

Mojibur Rahman writes on the contemporary child labour situation in South Asia and highlights the role of NGOs in combating child labour in Bangladesh and Nepal. Low level performance in securing 'universal primary education' for all has been claimed as a 'state failure' in the paper. At the same time he presents success stories of non-formal primary schooling of the NGOs in Bangladesh and Nepal.

Salahuddin Aminuzzaman, *Afroza Begum* & *F.R.M. Mortuza Huq* in their paper highlights the importance of Government-NGO collaboration in development management. The paper presents a scenario of health sector NGOs in Bangladesh and their prospects in operating collaborative health-care projects jointly with the Government. Based on the empirical findings of two collaborative health-care projects of two large NGOs and the Government of Bangladesh, the papers presents a set of strengths and weaknesses of such collaborative models.

A.K.M. Saifullah analyses the changes one of the World's largest NGOs, Bangladesh Rural Advancement Committee (BRAC) has undergone during the past decade. Responding to the pressures from donors to become more self-sufficient, BRAC has gone for various commercial ventures. In his article Saifullah assesses how this affects the original mission of the organisation.

2. MANAGERS, ADVOCATES, CRITICS AND OBJECTORS: DIVERSE STANDS ON DEVELOPMENT NGOS

Marko Ulvila

INTRODUCTION

The increase of official development aid flows to non-governmental organisations and relaxation of regulations regarding association in many Southern countries has resulted in a social change where more and more people both in the North and the South are engaged in very diverse development activities under a framework of NGOs. Non-governmental organisations are defined here, following Tvedt (1998), as organisation within the development aid channel that are institutionally separated from the state apparatus and are non-profit distributing.

The phenomenon has received attention from an increasing number of professionals engaged in research, evaluation and commentary. Several research monographs, edited volumes and special issues of academic journals have been devoted to the topic. The studies are almost as diverse as the field ranging from small evaluation reports to series of books coming out of long research project involving multi-disciplinary teams. Also the approach and the ideological standing of the authors varies greatly.

In this article I first discuss the history of the Northern NGOs involved in international activity. Then some of the important early writings on development NGOs are introduced. The last part of the article presents four approaches found in the literature to the issue with examples of recent texts. They are aid project management, neo-liberal advocacy, leftist critique and radical objection.

ORIGINS AND ACTIVITIES OF THE NGOS

The origins of the Western non-governmental organisations that are active in the areas now know as developing countries could be traced as far back as to the era of 'discoveries' when European travellers, often guided by Arabs, Asians and Africans, explored areas previously unknown to their civilisation. Along with the explorers there were representatives of the church. However, as the church and the state were not separated at that time the term non-governmental is not really appropriate. Nevertheless, missionary societies form unquestionably the first set of institutions that have evolved into several religiously oriented development NGOs of today.

The relations of the early missionary organisations with their home governments also set a pattern that is common even today. The missionary societies received subsidies from the colonial governments especially for their health and education activities. In return they accepted what they believed was benevolent colonialism and encouraged obedience to the rulers. During the independence movements that first took Latin America and later Asia and Africa the missionaries supported the legitimacy and desirability of colonial rule almost to the end. (Smith 1990, 28-29)

Another pattern of NGO activity was set by the establishment of the International Red Cross in the late 1850s in a response to the suffering of the victims in the War of Italian Succession. The movement spread fast to help war victims in other European and American countries. These societies became soon to be partially subsidised by their governments as they were found to be valuable instruments in caring for the wounded during war time. (Smith 1990, 30) Since then the suffering caused by war has prompted establishment of numerous other relief organisations. For example the Save the Children Fund of UK began in 1919 as a response to the Allied blockade of Germany, in the UK Oxford Committee for Famine Relief started in 1942, in the US Catholic Relief Services in 1943 and CARE in 1945 and in Denmark Mellenfolkelig Samwirke in 1994. (OECD 1988, 18) Besides providing relief to the public suffering from war, at times these NGOs have played an active role in the war efforts of the Western powers. For example in the Korean war major religious and secular NGOs, including Lutheran World Relief, provided food and clothes through the US Army. (Smith 1990, 51-52) After the Second World War and its aftermath practically all of these organisations have extended their activities to developing countries, especially to provide relief in conflict areas but also to conduct development projects elsewhere.

The late 19th century saw yet a third set of NGOs extending their activities overseas, namely secular educational and cultural organisations, trade unions and women's associations. By 1910 there were already 344 private nonprofit institutions in Europe and North America engaged in overseas activity. These organisations, again, received subsidies from their home government especially for work in their respective colonies. (Smith 1990, 31) These groups established a tradition which has later evolved into development NGOs working less on relief and more on development and partnership activities.

The organisations established by government or inter-governmental organisations could be considered a fourth pattern of NGO origins. One example is the UN Food and Agriculture Organisation's Freedom from Hunger campaign started in 1960 where national associations were established in a number of OECD countries. Some of them are still important today, for example the Comité francais contre la faim (founded in 1996) and Deutsche Welthungerhilfe (1963). (OECD 1988, 21) Another case are the Inter-America and Africa foundations set by the US government in the 1970s. (Smith 1990, 66)

As noted before, for centuries governments and their agencies have played important role in the operations of the development NGOs. In the era of development that begun after the Second World War the trend has augmented. Formal arrangements with governmental funding to development NGOs started in the United States in early 1950s. It was followed by Germany and Sweden in 1962, Australia, the Netherlands and Norway in 1965, Canada in 1968, and Finland in 1974. The Commission of European Communities set up its co-financing programme in 1975, United Kingdom in 1975 and France in 1977. (OECD 1988, 25)

To summarise, the main pattern of NGO activity and their relations with government was set already before the development era started in the early 1950s. These include missionary NGOs, war relief, secular developmental association and government initiated organisations. From the beginning, majority, if not all, of NGOs involved in the areas now know as developing countries have enjoyed considerable subsidies from their home government and in return supported their policies and presence in the Third World - even if they now are considered oppressive and violent.

EARLY STUDIES OF NGOS IN DEVELOPMENT

Some of the early studies of the 1980s on NGOs in development have set the scene for further debate on the issues. They have summarised some of the main reasons why NGOs have increasingly taken part in development co-operation efforts and assessed them against empirical studies. They have also set normative standards against which the NGOs are commonly analysed.

One of the first comprehensive studies on NGOs in development was done by Judith Tendler in 1982 for the United States Agency for International Development (AID). She was commissioned to review some 70 evaluations of the Private Voluntary Organisations (PVOs), as NGOs are called in the US, and to draw conclusions especially for further evaluation.

Tendler identified seven typical characteristics of NGOs that are considered as their comparative advantage in relation to state-to-state development assistance. According to these 'articles of faith' NGOs reach the poor, are participatory, apply process oriented methods, differ from the public sector by not being bureaucratic, corrupt, uncommitted and inefficient, are experimental and innovative, strengthen local institutions and work cost effectively. (Tendler 1982, 3-7)

In her analysis Tendler discusses four of the items in detail: participation, focus on the poor, relations with government and innovativenes. Her conclusion is that none of the articles of faith are validated in the evaluation material. On the contrary:

> "The work of PVOs may best be characterized as expanding or improving under existing techniques of delivery of public services. In many cases,

successful projects will involve a style that is top-down, though enlightened, and decentralized. Participation may or may not be involved. In certain cases, moreover, PVOs may be successful more as precursors to government than as innovators." (Tendler 1982, vii)

Interestingly, findings reverse to the Tendler's were soon presented by another study of the US NGOs. An OECD document on NGOs paraphrases a 1986 study on development effectiveness of private voluntary organisations prepared for the US Congress. It lists strengths of NGOs that have been "widely documented: ability to reach the rural poor in unserved areas, promotion of local participation, provision of low-cost services, use of adaptive and innovative technology and ability to maintain an independent status." The weaknesses include limited replicability, lack of financial sustainability and absence of programming strategies. (OECD 1988, 114)

This debate on the comparative advantage and opposing positions have featured centrally in the NGO literature ever since. At times the 'articles of faith' are endorsed and at times denied. In any case they continue to provide an important set of beliefs for both policy documents, public image and studies alike.

In 1987 David C. Korten published an influential article in a special NGO issue of the journal World Development analysing the past efforts of private voluntary organisation and providing suggestions for the future. Korten presented his views in a context where the current development crisis would have to meet with the challenge of democratisation. The necessary reforms involve complex organisational changes that the large official donors have little capability to address. Therefore the central leadership role must be assumed by NGOs with the potential to serve as catalysts of institutional and policy change. (Korten 1987, 145)

In the article Korten presented a categorisation of NGOs that has been widely referred to ever since. He called them the three generations of private voluntary development action:

> *First, Relief and welfare:* Relief activities are the origin also for many large welfare oriented NGOs.. "As these organizations brought their expertise to bear in non-disaster situations they gave birth to a first generation of private voluntary development assistance. As development strategy relief and welfare approaches offer little more than temporary alleviation of the symptoms of underdevelopment".

> *Second, Small-scale self-reliant local development:* Recognising the limitations of relief and welfare approaches, many NGOs undertook in the late 1970s community development activities such as preventive health, improved farming practices and local infrastructure. They stress local self-reliance sustained beyond the NGO assistance. Often the activities are parallel to those of the government in areas where government does not reach.

Third, Sustainable systems development: The focus of this approach is on facilitating sustainable changes in villages and sectors of NGO activity. The role is more catalytic rather than operational service-delivery. High levels of technical and strategic competence are required.

According to Korten, these strategic orientations often co-exist in an organisation. The generations do not therefore refer so much into organisations but to different programme approaches. (Korten 1987, 147-149)

In Korten's view a growing number of NGOs have realised the need to exert greater leadership in addressing dysfunctional aspects of the policy and institutional setting of the villages and sectors within which they work. This means moving to a third generation strategy in which the focus is on facilitating sustainable changes in these settings on a regional or even national basis. It will likely mean less direct involvement at village level for these particular NGOs, and more involvement with a variety of public and private organisations that control resources and policies that bear on local development. These may include local and national governments, private enterprises, other independent sector institutions etc. (Korten 1987, 149)

The analysis and suggestions of Korten has been very influential. For example, in one of the first OECD policy document on NGOs from 1988 it was referred to frequently. Nevertheless, it has also been criticised.[1] Terje Tvedt has pointed out that the framework "creates a mythical historical development from good to better, while neglecting much more important and real divisions and reducing the complexity of the NGO scent. It also ascribes to the channel as whole an agreement on normative thinking about the primary role of the NGOs the is untenable." (Tvedt 1998, 34)

FOUR APPROACHES TO NGOS

As all human action has political roots and consequences, also the NGO literature can be analysed according to their ideological standing. This task is made fairly easy by the fact that most of the writers on NGOs in development readily take stands and furnish advice for the policy makers in the government and organisations.

In the recent NGO literature four approaches to the NGO boom can be distinguished: aid project management, neo-liberal advocacy, leftist critique and radical objection.. The management perspective includes evaluation studies commissioned by the aid donor agencies whereby the activity is viewed in a project framework. Of the broader perspectives, the dominant one concurs with

---

[1] It should be added that there seems to be reverse transformation at place from more holistic and rooted approaches to relief and welfare operations. For example, in India many leaders of the the Gandhian holistic Sarwodaya movement have established foreign funded NGOs providing social services, including relief operations.

the neoliberal ideology of minimising the role of the state and liberalisation of economy. A counter current includes the critical examination that high-lights the positive role of the public sector and limitations of the NGOs, a traditional leftist view. The radical structuralist view consider the NGO expansion as part of the hegemonic capitalist system that should be objected. Below each approach is illustrated with a recent example.

Aid project management

By far most of the titles on development NGOs are evaluation reports commissioned by the donor agencies or the NGOs themselves as part of the project cycle or related reflections. While some of the studies do take broader issues into consideration, typically they operate on the project framework. Therefore common tasks are to observe if the planned project outputs have been realised, if the activity has been relevant to the intended beneficiaries, if the implementation has been cost-effective, if the project has had the desired effects and impact and if the changes are sustainable. Often some topical cross-cutting issues such as environment, gender, participation or such are studies as well. Typically the evaluation studies do not occupy themselves with broader questions such a origins of the growing NGO activity or the role of NGOs in regard to people's political organising or foreign policy objectives of the super-powers.

One example of the aid management approach is the synthesis study of NGO evaluations done for the Organisation for Economic Cooperation and Development's Development Assistance Committee's (OECD/DAC) Expert Group on Evaluation. The review encompassed 60 separate reports of 240 projects undertaken in 26 developing countries. The study was conducted under the leadership of Roger C. Riddell who has also co-authored a several major NGO evaluations for the donor agencies. (Riddell et al. 1997)

The evaluation synthesis study takes a very limited view on the question of NGOs. It does not touch on issues beyond a project framework such as NGO-government relations or economic and political trends affecting NGO activities. The firmest observation the study makes is that there is still a lot that needs to be studied - therefore giving more employment opportunities for the evaluation professionals.

There are four main issues on which the synthesis study comments based on the evaluation reports. According to the study, the assessment of impact on the lives of the poor varied considerably in the reports, ranging from significant benefits to little evidence of making much difference. However, all reports agree that even the best projects are insufficient to enable the beneficiaries to escape from poverty. Most projects examined are not financially sustainable, and the poorer the intended beneficiaries are the harder it is to reach financial sustainability. In the majority of the projects examined the benefits appeared to have exceeded the costs. Some studies praise NGOs for their innovativeness and others argue that there is little unique in their activities. (Riddell et al. 1997, 19-26)

When compared with the similar exercise done by Judith Tendler on the material from the United States in 1998 the narrow approach of the Riddell study becomes even more evident. Whereas Tendler distanced herself from the core aid discourse by grouping the assumptions about the NGOs into 'articles of faith' and critically examined if they can be substantiated from the evaluation reports Riddell is satisfied to assert himself within the simple aid discourse.

The cautious way of dealing with the subject matter can be partially be explained by the forum for which the synthesis study was made, the DAC Expert Group on Aid Evaluation. The OECD is one of the main forums for aid co-ordination among the northern donor countries. Besides being regulated by the courtesy of diplomatic conduct, the body is an important institution in the establishment of the hegemonic discourses on aid, and the restricted and uncritical view of NGOs fits well into the current trends.

Neoliberal advocacy

The current dominant paradigm and ideology in the world politics is often referred to as neoliberalism. Its essence are capitalist economy and liberal democratic polity. Earlier in this century the expansion of capitalism was arrested by communist and socialists rule in several countries both in the North and in the South. However in the early 1980s neoliberal ideology first gained upper hand in the North Atlantic countries and after the fall of the Soviet Union it has taken the world like a storm. The neoliberal shift has included liberalisation of trade and finances, strict control on government spending leading to cuts also in basic social services and the growth of the Third or volunteer sector. In developing countries the shift has often included restoration of multi-party democracy and relaxed regulations on association.

Given the hegemonic position of the neoliberal ideology it is easy to find authors on non-governmental organisations that readily agree with the views outlined below. One such example is a recent book 'Nongovernments: NGOs and the Political Development in the Third World' by Julia Fisher. (Fisher 1998)

Fisher's book is about the political and technical capacities of Third World NGOs and their relationships with their governments that in her view are growing and thus promoting sustainable development. The purpose of her book "is to present the considerable evidence that the cultivation of civil society, propelled by NGOs, can contribute to political development in the Third World." And political development she defines "as an interactive, public decision-making and learning process, within and between government and civil society, based on power creation and dispersion. This process leads to increasing individual and group autonomy from below and more responsiveness from above." (Fisher 1998, 21-29)

For Fisher the NGOs have proliferated because of the failure of the Southern governments to bring development to their people. According to Fisher, "the rise of Third World NGOs has coincided with the increasing inability of the nation-state to muddle through as it confronts the long-term consequences of its own ignorance, corruption, and lack of accountability." The governments have failed to meet the challenges of sustainable development, and especially the educated people have become aware of the gap between the desperate reality of the poor and what is possible. This has, according to Fisher, "also opened up unprecedented opportunities for NGOs not just to replace governments but to protest against them, influence them, and collaborate with them - in short, to radically alter the way that people in most of the world are governed." (Fisher 1998, 2-30)

Although Fisher recognises that the increased availability of international funding and the high level of unemployment among educated professionals has contributed to the proliferation of NGOs the main thrust of the argument is on the shortcoming of the governments. She states that "the inability of most regimes to raise living standards in local areas and the continued depletion of productive and natural resources by power elites set the political stage for the entrance of increasing numbers of NGOs." (Fisher 1998, 61)

Interestingly Fisher's book is totally silent about the political parties and elections, although her theme is political development. This is even more surprising given the fact that during the past two decades of NGO growth there has also been a vast transition from military and single party regimes to governments designated in multi-party elections. The reason is probably that in Fisher's opinion the 'ruling elites' that are running the bad governments of the South are also patronising the parties, whereas the NGOs represent a fresh force outside the local dominant power structures.

However, the fact that the work does not touch on the surmounting challenges posed by the global economy to the Third World governments and the people - such as worsening terms of trade, deepening foreign dept, and adaptation to the unfavourable WTO regime - is not surprising given the neoliberal thrust of the volume. Her idea of political development in isolation of political economy is typical to the genre.

In the preface to the book Fisher gives a hint of what she is about to undertake. She mentions that political development was part of the modernisation theory that fascinated her during her graduate studies and she retained the fascination even when later on the dependency theories "thought that the idea of political development was naive and ethnocentric". (Fisher 1998, xi) Naiveté can certainly be considered a characteristic of her analysis, and there is no shortage of ethnocentrism either. When defining NGOs she includes many kind of grassroots organisations and their support institutions, but "under conservative, authoritarian Arab regimes, most voluntary organizations are traditional charities, not NGOs." (Fisher 1998, 59) NGOs, for Fisher, are those which promote values dear to herself, whereas other kind of associations must be excluded from the purview.

Leftist critique

In the NGO literature there is also a critical trend which does not take the mainstream assumptions for granted but looks behind them for more tenable explanation of the phenomenon. Typically a critical study first presents the prevailing assumptions about the NGOs and then scrutinises them against empirical data. The example here is the monograph 'Angels of Mercy or Development Diplomats: NGOs and Foreign Aid' by Terje Tvedt. (Tvedt 1998)

First Tvedt attempts to bring clarity into the definition of NGOs. He observes that a basic problem with many a classification is that they are based on normative judgements - defining NGOs as having some positive but ambiguous characteristics such as self-reliance, voluntarism, popular membership base etc. The aim of such criteria is often to distinguish the good and fundable NGOs from the bad ones. However, for research purposes this is not useful because the so called 'bad NGOs' are also important part of the phenomenon. Therefore Tvedt defines NGOs operationally as "organisations within the aid channel that are institutionally separated from the state apparatus and are non-profit distributing". (Tvedt 1998, 12-36)

One of the main points of Tvedt is to challenge the explanations that attribute the growth of NGOs to market and government failures. One such is the public goods theory whereby the existence of NGOs is reasoned as a way to satisfy the residual unsatisfied demand for public goods in society. Where a significant minority wants a public good for which there is no majority support, the government cannot help and NGOs step in. Another related theory is the contract failure theory which explains the popularity of NGOs by people's trust on them rather than market producers. (Tvedt 1998, 41-42)

According to Tvedt there is no empirical support to these theories because most of the NGOs operate with official development assistance funds provided by the donor governments. As the funding to NGOs in the North and conducive environment to their activities in the South are deliberate acts by the government it is not meaningful to explain the raise of NGOs as a response to the failures of the governments. Such theories confuse the comprehension of the concrete historical development of the politico-economic context in which these organisations have mushroomed.

> To explain the growth of NGOs in these four countries by regarding them as
> a societal response to internal market or state failures is not very helpful.
> Rather, the majority of local NGOs have emerged as a response, not to
> internal conditions, but to the growth in political and financial initiatives on

the part of the donor community and the ongoing competition among donors for suitable and good local partners. (Tvedt 1998, 53)

Therefore Tvedt proposes that development NGOs must not be analysed within a national, third-sector perspective, but rather as an outcome of complicated processes where factors like international ideological trends, donor policies and NGO agendas interact with national historical and cultural conditions in complex ways. By combining a national-style approach, where the organisational structure and landscape in a particular country are seen as a reflection of its cultural and historical characteristics, with an international social system approach the complex development processes shaping the NGO scene in the aid area can be taken properly into account. Analysis of the NGO sector should therefore rather be looked upon as one social system, and a social system of a particular kind. It is a global system, donor-led but with a great number of supporters in the developing countries. The development NGOs as an international social system is characterised by the flow of development assistance funding, shared language and symbolic order, and the ideal-type project model where NGO articulates the needs of the poor, receives funding, implements the activity and evaluates it. (Tvedt 1998, 66-90)

Approaching the questions of development NGOs from the international social system approach and using was empirical material from Norway Tvedt makes observations about the idea of NGOs having comparative advantage vis-a-vis the governments and about the 'articles of faith' on NGO superioirity. According to Tvedt there has not been any convincing study to substantiate this 'list of dogmas', and the whole concept of comparative advantage is hardly meaningful because the state and NGOs are so different by their orientation and by the instruments of action. Actually the strength of the NGOs could in fact be the comparative disadvantage in operational terms, their commitment to values that might make them less efficient or competitive. (Tvedt 1998, 128-136)

> To sum up: NGOs in development do not function in any specific way. They do not have important common characteristics or potentials, apart from three: They receive money from public donors, they are formally independent and they are non-profit distributing. Their roles in societies vary tremendously, however. It is therefore more useful to analyse how different organiszations have played and are playing different social, political and cultural roles in different contexts, than to try to summarize general characteristics. ... NGOs do not have the general comparative advantages the NGO language and official documents ascribe to them. This term, taken from neo-classical economic theory, is not useful in the aid context and blurs empirical understanding and assessment. (Tvedt 1998, 156)

The critical study of NGOs recognises the fact that NGOs do not work in isolation but are very much related to the development aid funding regime ruled by the northern donor government. There are national differences both in the

North and the South which creates different kind of NGO activity, but the international social system is dominant one. Although the critical approach links the NGOs to the broader aid framework it does not extend its analysis to wider political economy.

Radical objection

A less articulated but yet important approach to the NGOs is that of the radical structuralism. This view sees NGOs as unnecessary or even detrimental element in a developing society. Prior to the collapse of the Soviet Union and its model of communist development, NGOs were not encouraged, or even tolerated, in many developing countries. Since the beginning of the 1990's and the emergence of the unchallenged position of the neoliberal order the radical structuralist view of NGOs has become fairly marginal. It is, however, worth presenting here because although the Soviet model collapsed it did not necessarily invalidate the radical strucutralist critique of capitalism. It is only the hegemonic view that there are no alternatives to capitalist/neoliberal state of affairs that considers the radical structuralist critique outdated and irrelevant.

As there is no monograph or edited volume on the radical structuralist critique of the development NGOs an article of Yash Tandon is presented here as an example. [2]

Drawing on African experience Tandon emphasises the context in which the current NGO boom exists. Since the 1980's Africa has witnessed falling standard of living since. According to him the reasons are not civil strife, ethnic wars or the lack of democracy and transparency but the lack of control Africans have over their own resources. Land is not always owned by Africans or the products of the land are either controlled by transnational corporations or traded in the world market at prices below their real value. In the post-cold war era the Western countries want to retain their powers and sell their ideas to the South. Poor are seen as an enemy from which the white Christian Western nations protect themselves by erecting immigration barriers against the people of colour. Given the weakness of the African leadership the Western powers are openly advocating direct intervention in Africa's internal affairs. The development aid is used as a sanction and new discourse is of management of Africa's politics and economics. The West is laying down the instrumentalities and modalities of a new technocratic order in Africa. (Tandon 1996, 179-182)

In this context Tandon sees the NGOs are the advanced guard of the new era of Africa's recolonisation. They play a similar role to the missionaries in the colonial times where they neutralised the ideological defences of colonised

---

[2] Another set of the contemporary radical structuralist critique of NGOs are the positions of Communist groups engaged in armed struggle in South Asia, such as the Communist Party of Nepal (Maoists) or the People's War Group in Andrha Pradesh, India. These writings are mainly published in vernacular languages in local press.

peoples and thus prepared the ground for colonial occupation. Today the NGOs have four kinds of detrimental roles:

(i)   diversionary: drawing attention away from the real causes of Africa's poverty,

(ii)   ideological: professing the universality of Western values of democracy, human rights, feminism and environmentalism; brainwashing a section of the middle class,

(iii)   pacification of people suffering from the effects of structural adjustment, subverting African grassroots and radical critique of the imperial project,

(iv)   destructive of African institutions of education, traditional agriculture, traditional healing and health practices and governance. (Tandon 1996, 182-183)

The radical structuralist view on the NGOs thus pays attention not to projects or to development aid in general, but the structure of international economy and political power. In this context development aid is seen as self-serving programme of the donor countries and NGOs as its extension. Except for the few NGOs struggling on these broader issues the rest is seen as harmful for liberation of the people and the nations if the Third World.

CONCLUSIONS

Although developmental non-governmental organisations is often considered a new phenomenon, they have predecessors dating all the way to colonial times. In fact the basic patterns of the NGOs and their relations with the Northern governments were well established before the 'era of development' began in post World-War-II international relations and political economy. It is important to keep this historical perspective in mind when analysing the present day NGOs, because the old patterns of interaction between the Northern dominant governments and their NGOs have many similarities today.

The four approaches to development NGOs presented here could provide some assistance for anybody interested in reviewing the literature on the theme. The ideological classification used here is by no means the only viable one, and other analysis needs to be made for obtaining a more comprehensive picture.

REFERENCES

Fisher, Julie (1998) *Nongovernments: NGOs and the Political Development of the Third World*. West Hartford: Kumarian Press.

Korten, David C. (1987) Third Generation NGO Strategies: A Key to People-centered Development. *World Development*, Vol 15, Supplement Autumn, 1987 145-159.

OECD (1988) *Voluntary Aid for Development: The Role of Non-Governmental Organisations*. Paris: Organisation for Economic Co-operation and Development.

Riddell, Roger C. et al (1997) *Searching for Impact and Methods: NGO Evaluation Synthesis Study*. A Report prepared for the OECD/DAC Expert Group on Evaluation. By Roger C. Riddel, Stein-Erik Kruse, Timo Kyllönen, Satu Ojanperä and Jean-Louis Vieljus. Helsinki: Ministry for Foreign Affairs, Department for International Development Cooperation.

Smith, Brian H. (1990) *More than Altruism: the Politics of Private Foreign Aid*. Princeton: Princeton University Press.

Tendler, Judith (1982) *Turning Private Voluntary Organizations Into Development Agencies: Questions for Evaluation*. AID Program Evaluation Discussion Paper No 12. Washington DC: U.S. Agency for International Development.

Tandon, Yash (1996) An African Perspective. In Sogge, David (ed) *Compassion & Calculation: The Business of Private Foreign Aid*. London: Pluto Press.

Tvedt, Terje (1998) *Angels of Mercy or Development Diplomats: NGOs and Foreign Aid*. Oxford: James Currey.

3. SUSTAINABILITY OF NGO-LED DEVELOPMENT PROJECTS: LESSONS FROM SOUTH ASIA

Farhad Hossain

INTRODUCTION

The role of Non-Governmental Organisations (NGOs) in managing development initiatives in developing countries has been very central in contemporary development aid discourse. The reasons for the emergence of development NGOs since the 1970s are several. Among them 'market failure' and 'government failure' are considered the leading ones in developing countries. (Anheier & Seibel 1990, 1) Scholars argue that this growth of NGOs is a reflection of dissatisfaction with both state and market. On the other hand, the use of NGOs has been consistent with both the New Right aid policies of governments in the USA and UK and the 'alternative' aid policies of the consciences of the donor community in the Nordic countries and the Netherlands. (Hulme 1994, 251 & 265) The restructuring policies of the World Bank and other influential donor institutions (e.g. in OECD countries) led to a planned reduction of the role of the state in developing countries and increased space for development NGOs. (Tvedt 1998, 62)

However, sustainability of NGO-led development initiatives are being questioned. The present paper discusses the issue of sustainability of the NGO-led development projects only in Bangladesh and Nepal as a representative model from South Asia. The paper has been prepared based on the empirical findings of recent research works on the development programmes in central, northern, & north-eastern part of Bangladesh (Hossain 1998b; Hossain & Ulvila & Khan 1999; Ulvila & Saifullah & Hossain 2000) and mid-western & central part of Nepal (Hossain 1998b; Hossain & Dhakal 1999; Dhakal & Hossain 1999). South Asia's development scenario has common elements and is shared by most of the states in the region – however findings of this study should not broadly be generalised.

DEVELOPMENT AND NGOS

Comparative advantage of NGOs is widely claimed in development aid literature. Development projects, run by NGOs are assumed as flexible, innovative, participatory, cost-effective and directed to the poor. For the donors, one of the major reasons for the increasing use of NGOs in developmental activities is to find an alternative and better channel for development aid. The aim of this search, as the donors often argue, is to pluralise the actors or stakeholders involved in development activities so that the 'poorest of the poor' could be reached more effectively, by bypassing the oligarchic state structure of most of the developing countries. Thus disappointment and criticism with public sector performance, in both donor and recipient countries, have had an important impact on this development. From a more general perspective the issue is also related to the continuously declining situation of third world development, characterised by recurrent economic crises, population growth, environmental degradation, poor agricultural and industrial production, growing corruption, bureaucratic complexities, inadequate policies, lack of democratic exercise in domestic politics, and the politics of debt crisis in developing countries. As a reaction to this general context, the western donor countries and agencies are seeking better ways to implement their policies by considering the comparative advantages and disadvantages of the organisations that are involved in this process. (Mälkiä & Hossain 1998, 28)

Disappointment with public sector performance has played an important role in recent developments. While public sector activities continue to be heavily criticised for having contributed much to the present problematic situation in many developing countries, NGOs are receiving much credit and gaining a greater status in development work. Whereas disappointment with official government programs and projects is growing, the NGOs have gained such prominence that development transfers through these types of organisations have become more or less obvious from the donors' point of view (see e.g. Anheier 1990). For example in Norway, in the beginning of the 1990s the share of bilateral aid to NGOs was 25 per cent, with the percentage continuing to increase (Tvedt 1995, i). In the United States the government has announced that in future it is going to channel about 40 per cent of its development assistance through NGOs (United Nations 1995, 2). And, according to a calculation (Fowler 1992, 17), the value of total resources from NGOs to the third world countries accounts for about 15 per cent of total overseas development assistance.

In contrast to official development agencies, the non-governmental organisations are believed to have fewer overhead costs, to rely less on bureaucratic procedures, and to be less subject to political constraints (e.g. Anheier 1990). All these conventional believes and practices among the donor community have contributed in the rise of NGOs globally. The rise of NGOs in South Asia is also directly linked to this new aid practice in world development.

SOUTH ASIAN DEVELOPMENT SCENARIO

Despite the recent economic advances in many parts of Asia, South Asia remained economically poor and infrastructurally vulnerable. South Asia covers an area of about 4.6 million square kilometres, which is only 3.31 per cent of the total land mass in the world. In mid-1990, the total population of South Asia was estimated at 1130 million, that is roughly 1/5th of the human race – which was rapidly growing. During the eighties, the population growth rate in South Asia was 2.4 per cent as against 0.8 per cent for the industrialised world. Among the one billion poorest people in the world, 35 per cent lives in South Asia -- in terms of 'quality of life' indicates such as infant mortality per 1000 population, life expectancy, literacy, etc., South Asia's performance remained generally poor. (see for details Khan 1990; Siddique 1992; Quibria 1994)

As a result, South Asia has been the home of numerous development projects, supported by the OECD donor countries and agencies over the decades. Health care and education projects of Christian missionary organisations have a long tradition also in South Asia – however the modern NGO-led development projects began from the beginning of the 1970s. NGOs in South Asia are believed to succeeded in bringing about relevant and effective institutional changes at the grass-roots level to facilitate implementation of need-based development efforts to improve the quality of life of the rural poor. The conventional paradigm, followed by the government, has not, in fact, shown much success in ameliorating the poverty of the rural people who constitute the bulk of the population in most of the South Asian countries. The process of centralised planning and the top-down implementation of programmes through the rigid, non-responsive bureaucratic apparatus, as conceived in such paradigm, fail to accommodate the needs and priorities of the rural poor. In fact, most of the resources provided by the government tend to gravitate towards the richer section of the population having power and political patronage. Many of the macro policy-reforms, made by the government from time to time with a view to benefiting the poor, have failed to achieve desired successes, primarily because of the non-existence of appropriate institutions to execute such reforms at the grass-roots level. It is here that NGOs are thought to play an important role in complementing the government efforts through developing appropriate institutions and concomitant value-systems. (Huda 1987, 1)

Since 1970s, the OECD donors have increasingly been involving NGOs in development management. However, the gap between the rich and the poor remained more or less unchanged throughout developing Asia.

Research suggests (see e.g. Kalimullah 1990, 171) that also the experience of NGO led development has so far been disappointing in developing countries despite the donors' growing interest to involve them in their development mission. Several decades have passed and NGOs have had limited success, having failed largely in their efforts to reduce rural poverty by any significant amount. The idea, for example, that NGOs have the comparative advantage that they are generally assumed to have in the literature on NGOs in development, has been falsified. (Tvedt 1997, 1) South Asia is going to experience this disappointment if the actors are not well aware in advance about the shortcomings of this sector and do not try to evaluate, learn and overcome these shortcomings.

SUSTAINABILITY OF NGO-LED DEVELOPMENT PROJECTS: ANALYSIS FROM SELECTED CASE STUDIES FROM BANGLADESH AND NEPAL

Riddel et al (1995, 56) argues that to *review and assess* all initiatives funded against the achievement of sustainability do not necessarily mean that the future financial or institutional sustainability should in all cases be a *necessary* requirement for funding discrete projects or programmes. In particular, financial and institutional sustainability need to be pursued only on condition that, especially for the poor and where basic needs or services are being provided, the quality of, and access to, the basic goods or service provided will not be radically compromised. Where the goods or service provided is considered essential to the basic well-being of the beneficiaries, and where alternative funding cannot be found, the inability to achieve either financial or institutional sustainability should not constitute an impediment to funding such NGO initiatives.

A development programme is considered sustainable when it is able to deliver an appropriate level of benefits for an extended period of time after major financial, managerial, and technical assistance from an external donor is terminated. (OECD 1989, 13) OECD compendium of evaluation experience added some of the key points (OECD 1989, 7) of this definition. In the light of the compendium, some of the studied NGO-led development programmes in northern & north-eastern part of Bangladesh (Hossain 1998b; Hossain & Ulvila & Khan 1999; Ulvila & Saifullah & Hossain 2000) and mid-western & central part of Nepal (Hossain 1998b; Hossain & Dhakal 1999; Dhakal & Hossain 1999) could be analysed as follows:

One key issue of assessing sustainability is to asses the sustaining flow of benefits – the results or impact of a programme – that are relevant to a developing country's priority needs and the interest of decision-makers and beneficiaries. (OECD 1989, 7) Most of the NGO-led development programmes in Bangladesh and Nepal might have an impact on the lives of the people with a degree of benefits. Education projects, microcredit finance, community health care, awareness creation, etc. activities have a positive impact and people get benefit from these programmes. However, most of the NGO-run programmes has already been practised earlier by several other public organisations in the region – thus in present day NGO programmes are generally overlapping among them and also with other public organisations. There exists a lack of co-operation and co-ordination in operating development initiatives. Microcredit finance, nonformal primary education, social forestry, etc. programmes of few NGOs, has no doubt, made some success in the region. However, very little of the NGO development approach, in general, is innovative, cost-effective and flexible -- however participation of the people specially from the local community exists with good spirit. The level of participation and flexibility exists in NGO sector are only in the given environment, e.g. decided mostly by the NGO leaders and practised by the target groups. The NGO programmes are not generally designed specially by the countries leading policy makers or have not been designed to fulfil the governments prior sectors. However, several elements of NGO programme have some importance to the government policy makers but the interest of the governments is not that strong that they would undertake the NGO-led development projects if the NGOs become unable to run their programmes due to the unavailability of foreign aid. Most of the NGOs in Bangladesh and Nepal found to work with a degree of isolation from the government offices, e.g. with the local government institutes. Extreme dependency on and availability of foreign aid also keeps the NGO leaders' attention away from mobilising local resources, building effective partnership with the government institutions – which would have a long sustained impact of NGO activities in the region. Rather most of the NGO programmes were designed to make them adoptive and acceptable to the donors' policy -- a conventional practice in NGO sector to attract foreign aid – many of these programmes might not share the priority needs of the government development plans.

In order to achieve sustainable benefits and maintain supporting activities and institutions development interventions and projects should be specific. (OECD 1989, 7) Most of the NGOs are not involved only one specific project in Bangladesh and Nepal, rather they are practising an 'all-sector' approach in their development intervention. It does not look like that the development intervention of the NGOs would support or maintain the created institutions if foreign support is withdrawn. Limiting their activities, e.g. in education, or in health care, or in credit, etc. would help the NGOs to strengthen their village institutions. NGOs are not only involving themselves in many sectors, they are also expanding their activities in many regions in the country (e.g. several districts in a country) rather working in a specific geographical area. Except few large NGOs in the region most of the NGOs with their present professional knowledge and management capacity may gradually fail to deliver benefits to the poor if they involve themselves in numerous sectors of development and in various regions – this also might weaken NGOs and their institutions.

In assessing sustainability the 'appropriate level of benefits' and the 'extended period of time' of the OECD (1989) definition should also be defined in each instance by taking into account the country's development objectives, the initial investment and recurrent costs and the creation of a permanent institutional capacity. It is difficult to assess the 'appropriate level of benefits' of a development initiative in countries like Bangladesh and Nepal. Materialistically, as an example, Nepal might lack a lot, as UNDP ranks it in Human Development Index as 148th among 163 countries in the world. (UNDP 1998, 32) The present per capita income of Nepal is only USD 210 (Nepal South Asia Center 1998, 13). However the average Nepali do not find themselves poor as long as they do not compare themselves with industrially rich countries. Nepali Scholar Dor Bahadur Bista puts it like this:

> Nepal has historically been self-sufficient and the idea of foreign assistance is a new one. Nepalis may be poor by international standard but the Nepali peasants are self-sufficient and largely content. Because of their isolation from international affairs, Nepalis had no idea that they were relatively impoverished until a few decades ago. With an increasing awareness of the relative affluence of the western world and other benefits of modern technology a desire for a change in the economic base of the country has been felt. Along with it has also increased the awareness of being the poorest country of the world. This is being to destroy the gracefulness, charm, generosity and hospitality even among the rural people. So the improved condition of Nepal in statistical terms is not necessarily all positive. People are paying their prices in terms of some positive human values which once lost will not be that easy to reinstate for generations to come. (Bista 1994, 133)

Therefore, the dilemma of the above mentioned 'dual notion' of presenting the economic status of Nepal like many developing countries make it more difficult to determine the 'appropriate level of benefits'. However, after considering the socio-economic standard in Bangladesh and Nepal it could be said that: the benefit (in healthcare, education, etc.) people receive from NGOs seemed to be quite appropriate, at least it has relevance to the need of the poor. Most of the NGOs in the region were not found to follow any specific time table in implementing their development programmes. The time frame practise seems open-ended -- as long as foreign aid is available for the multipurpose & multisectoral projects. Presently, some of the foreign donors are trying to encourage sustainability of their supported projects – but the NGOs find it too late to encourage them in sustaining their activities, as the phase-out period has officially expired or scheduled to the end soon. (Chaudhari H. 1999 - interview) They need more time to begin with the initiatives to make their projects sustainable. (Rokeya 1996 - interview)

The termination of major external assistance assumes the developing country will provide the financial, technical and managerial resources required to sustain the programme. Continuing relations with external technical groups and supplementary financing of commodities may often be desirable. (OECD 1989, 7) Most of the government officials provided the insight that NGOs have mostly been developing their activities without consultation and co-operation with them. Therefore there is not any chance that the local government or the central government authorities would undertake NGO-led development projects and provide the financial, technical and managerial resources required to sustain their programmes. Social Welfare Council (SWC) or the Government in Nepal do not have any plan to provide the financial, technical and managerial resources required to sustain NGO programme, if foreign funding is withdrawn. (Pokharel 1999 - interview) In Bangladesh the government response would be the same. It should also be mentioned that some NGOs limits its activities among specific communities and the governments are working with people from every walk of life. Undertaking such NGO activities, providing services only to certain communities in a region by ignoring the general poor could not be justified – as the poor are many and poverty does not follow any border or does not concern only one community among the poor.

The whole program of development NGOs in Bangladesh and Nepal, largely (if not totally) depended on foreign funding. The present statistics show that 99.97% of the total annual funding of a NGO in Nepal comes from the external donors (Chaudhari 1998, 14). The present activities of most of the NGOs e.g. running of literacy class, microcredit, health, etc. services are not run with the local resources. It was found that the alternative source of generating resources to run the activities were not yet developed – that is the case for most of the NGOs. Phasing down or phasing out of the development programs or even decreasing the salaried personnel could raise questions: What would be the level of sustainability if many of the employees (who did not take other employment for their career) would lose their employment?

FACTORS AFFECTING SUSTAINABILITY: PERSPECTIVES FROM BANGLADESH AND NEPAL

Government Policies

Since the independence, NGOs have become an integral part of the institutional framework of the development management in Bangladesh. Since the 1970s, there has been a spectacular growth of NGOs in number and the NGOs have extended their programme coverage from relief and rehabilitation to education, health, human & economic development, gender equality and environment. NGOs are also increasingly becoming involved in some critical areas like human rights watch-dog, policy analysis think tank, etc. (Aminuzzaman 1994, 2). During recent years, the NGOs have entered into an operational arena which has traditionally been the 'exclusive domain' of the government or public sector. As a matter of fact, given its operational efficiency, experienced manpower, the NGOs, in effect are penetrating into that exclusive ground with increasing forces (University of Dhaka 1994, 1). The significance of the NGOs involved in the overall development programmes in Bangladesh could be seen from the pattern of inflow of foreign resources to the sector. The proportion of total foreign aid to Bangladesh disbursed through NGOs was already about one percent in 1972-73 (Abed et al. 1984 cited in Aminuzzaman 1998). During the mid eighties, on an average about 16 percent of the total foreign aid inflow was mediated through the

NGOs. At present about 20 percent of the foreign aid flow to the country is channelled through NGOs. As a result of the supportive government policy, by the year 1994, a little more than 14000 NGOs were registered with Department of Social Welfare, Ministry of Women and Children Affairs and NGO Affairs Bureau in Bangladesh (Aminuzzaman 1994). Another statistics shows that the proportion of total foreign aid to Bangladesh disbursed through NGOs was about 1 per cent only in 1972-73 which by the end of FY 1986-87, reached to 17.4 per cent. (Aminuzzaman & Begum 2000, 111) Certainly the percent has increased further over the years.

The policy of the Government of Nepal concerning NGOs has become relatively supportive after 1990. The number of NGOs has been doubling in each recent year. (Hossain 1998, 108-113) The Eighth Plan (1992-97) also supported the growth of NGOs in Nepal. The Ninth Plan (1997-2002) also has taken NGOs as development partners targeted to make the activities more effective creating an environment for conducting their activities in a co-ordinated manner. (National Planning Commission 1997, 46)

Apart from enjoying a degree of liberal support from the Governments the NGOs could not build an effective partnership with the government and their programmes remained largely unsustainable (Pokharel 1999). The NGO programmes remained largely isolated from the government programmes at field level and NGO leaders have a tendency to compete rather than co-operate with the government. Thus they are lacking the prospect to sustain their activities through the governments.

Management Capacity

Except few exceptions, the overall managerial capacity of the public and private institutes are not very good in South Asia. (Pokharel 1999 - interview) Therefore, the governments gave space for NGOs in the countries' development efforts with an expectation that NGOs would do better in their management practice. Theoretically this is also the justification of this special sector to exist. However, except for few NGOs, the managerial capacity of the NGO sector in Nepal remained largely backward (Pokharel 1999 - interview) and the case in Bangladesh is also the same (Ahmed 1996 - interview). The International Institute of Rural Reconstruction also states (IIRR 93-2501EI) that most of the NGOs exercise leadership without basic management skills. In countries like Bangladesh and Nepal NGO leaders consider their leadership practice charismatic. Also the linkage with the foreign donors adds a degree of respect to the charismatic style of leadership – which more or less exists due to the professional & financial dependency of the lower level personnel or field workers of NGOs and its target groups. None challenge the leader and his/her managerial skill in effective management – although the leaders have very little management skill. In general, NGO leadership might have some syndrome of this kind. However the NGO leaders remained ambitious about their capacity in the region. (see e.g. Hossain 2000, 80) As a result, the organisations remain unsustainable with its managerial practices – also due to the fact that the external and internal linkages of NGO programmes are not properly managed.

Organisation

Very often the organisational structure of NGOs is weak with the problems of unclear role, weak administration and poor communication. They put emphasis on rapid responses rather than long-term solutions. (IIRR 93-2501EI) In South Asia NGOs are not peoples' democratic organisations -- at least this is the case with the NGOs in Bangladesh and Nepal. Usually they are run by an executive committee (or a board), represents a limited number of general members and often they are not the target group. The development programmes of NGOs are not run by membership subscriptions – rather these programmes almost totally depend on foreign aid provided by external donor agencies. Thus these organisations remain largely vulnerable to the donor in deciding their development plans. Even the NGO executives are not confident that their organisations would run if donors withdraw their money. Therefore, it is not likely that these organisations would be sustainable with the present spirit if foreign money stops.

Local participation

Participation must be seen as an exercise of giving the rural poor the means to have a direct involvement in development projects (Oakley and Marsden 1990, 64). In the case of NGOs, although in the programme level the local community might have participation, the participation could not be considered 'direct', as it is limited only to the implementation period. Usually all 'rural poor' are not equally considered in NGO programme, rather their programme is mainly designed for specific communities. In practice a huge number of poor outside the community can not enjoy the services although they have a similar socio-economic status like the served ones. Usually economic participation of the clients in microcredit programmes is good but not enough to make the programmes sustainable if external donation stops. Their projects are not giving possibilities to the villagers for meaningful participation (e.g. in decision making, planning, etc.) rather limiting the participation only in receiving services. Improved initiative to strengthen the poors income would give NGOs a possibility to sustain their activities by their clients.

Financial factors

Community contribution to the initiative should not be expected much due to the overall socio-economic condition in developing countries. Fund-raising capabilities and arrangements should be improved for local community participation, but in practice often the raised fund does not contribute much to the overall cost of the project. As NGOs are dealing with people from the poorer segment of society, therefore provision concerning initiating users' fee might exclude the poor from the project. And the project aim could gradually be jeopardised by the middle class and the richer section of the society. Therefore improving the financial capacity of the poor to buy services could be considered by the operating NGOs in advance. (OECD 1989) Community contribution is not generally sought by NGOs in Bangladesh and Nepal. Local fund-raising initiative found largely absent or very minimum for the project costs and initiatives towards local resource mobilisation are also poor. It might be that fund-raising in villages in the region will not might be an effective approach. However, there exists ample opportunities to mobilise local resources through initiating income generating activities with the assistance of the poor, e.g. co-operative farming, goat rearing, poultry, dairy, etc. as the NGOs find appropriate in the areas they operate.

Technological factors

Depending on the project the overall technological competence of the poor are not advanced, if not absent. Communities' capability of operating and maintaining the technology in indigenous sectors e.g. agriculture, fisheries, rural transportation, etc. is good. Usually the project operating NGO and the donors select the types (e.g. health, agriculture, empowerment, advocacy, etc.) of the project or project services in advance. The target group has very little chance in technology selection. Therefore, the role in technology selection should be discussed in advance among the donors, NGOs, and the project beneficiaries. Acceptance of technology by the target groups very much depends on the provision of prior consultation with them. At the same time, use and improvement of local technology should also be considered. (OECD 1989) Services provided by most of the NGOs in Bangladesh and Nepal do not include sophisticated technologies. Agricultural support to the villagers may include providing high yielding varieties of vegetable seeds – which has probably been provided by many government and private agencies in the villages. Distributing contraceptive materials, e.g. condoms, tablets do not require advanced technologies. Missionary organisations were found managing the project related technologies well due to presence of their expatriate workers. Some 12 traditional wells were established by a NGO in Nepal were not managed and maintained properly – rather it was seemingly endangering the children of the village as the wells were found without any cover – children may accidentally fall down to these wells. At the same time these open wells are very vulnerable to contamination. Having knowledge in technology using might be more important that the technological inventions in these cases.

Most of the village poor are not in a position to select their technologies they needs. This is due to their traditional approach towards life and the process of production they practised over the centuries. Thus in future, NGOs should not expect much in technology selection from the villagers – rather they should encourage the existing appropriate technologies and new technologies what would have a sustainable use by the villagers and a sustainable effect on the local progress.

Socio-cultural factors

In transitional societies socio-cultural factors may affect the sustainable progress of the society – especially where there exists competition between the traditional practices and modern way of life (see for details Bista 1994) – what is also present in Bangladesh, Nepal and elsewhere in South Asia.

In many societies, women participation in development is weak due to several cultural and economic factors. While economic growth in overall Asia has admittedly led to some gains for a significant minority of women, the overall plight of Asian women remains unsatisfactory and unaddressed. Despite the ascendancy of some prime ministers and presidents in the region. (Asian Development Bank 1994, 2) Bangladesh and Nepal are not exceptions. However, in NGO-led development projects' participation of women in development is on the increase – although they are not yet recognised as the mainstream of the economic life rather village women found very active in agricultural production in the region. NGOs could ensure further women participation in their projects. Their participation should be built in such a way so that disadvantaged women can feel that their participation is meaningful for them and for the project. Only symbolic participation does not contribute to a good level of project performance.

Excessive use of alcohol (raksi) among men is common in some Nepali villages – which keeps them away from the economic production and progress. Patriarchal families are common in the region – therefore excessive use of alcohol by male members let the family fall in disastrous condition in Nepal. NGOs could aware the community about the bad affect of the alcohol to sustain the progress of the village.

Finally, good development initiatives by good NGOs, no doubt, deserve appreciation. NGOs could have better partnerships by developing a co-ordinated approach with other public and private agencies working in the region. It would avoid problems of overlapping with other agencies; would help NGOs to avoid the high service costs; and provide a possibility of sustaining their programmes with the assistance from other local agencies, especially from the government ones. At present, the South Asian villagers depend on several public, private, and non-profit institutions for their everyday affairs. These agencies have also been playing a significant role to their lives over the decades. Through the passage of time many institutions (stated earlier) among them remained sustainable with their existence and services. Compare to them the NGOs are the new ones in the region – started their operation only since the 1970s in Bangladesh and 1990s in Nepal. Thus it is the NGOs who to learn and understand the essence of sustainability of other agencies in the region in order to make their own initiatives more sustainable.

SUSTAINABILITY OF DEVELOPMENT INITIATIVES: THE DONOR, THE RECIPIENT AND THE OPERATING NGOS

The central concept of this chapter is the **sustainability of NGO-led development initiatives / projects**. The previous analysis on sustainability might have some complex elements and does not make the central concept easier for the community to understand. For analytical purposes, three influential factors have been identified that affects the sustainability of NGO-led development projects. In practice, three factors, i.e. (Hossain 1998b): **a.** *the overall and particular work environment of the NGOs in the target country;* **b.** *policy and the degree of commitment of the donors concerning NGOs;* and **c.** *the overall management capacity of the operating NGOs;* are the most influential factors, affect the sustainability of NGO-led development projects. A proper analysis on the policy & commitment of the **donor;** the overall & particular **environment** of the project in the target country; and an analysis of the administrative capacity of the concerned **NGOs** would help to assess the sustainability of NGO-led development projects.

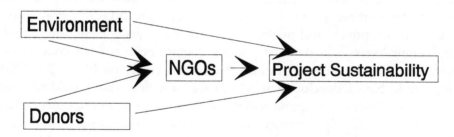

Examination and analysis of **the environment** where NGOs are operating their projects are important for the successful completion of the project. Particularly, the working environment of the NGOs in the concerned country should be examined whether government policies are supportive towards their activities or not.

Examination and analysis of the position of the official **donors and donor NGOs** are important. Their policies at home and the strength, commitment, etc. for development projects abroad should be studied in analysing the sustainability of the development projects.

Examination and analysis of **Management capacity of the operating NGOs** particularly, their development initiatives or projects should be made. For example the organisation, local participation e.g. scope of management and organisational factors, managerial leadership, development of organisational capabilities, etc. should properly be studied.

FINAL FINDINGS AND THE CONCLUDING REMARKS

From the above discussions it could be mentioned that sustainability of NGO-led development depends on certain factors and these factors are interdependent. Apart from this, we should also view NGOs as part of a larger global economic and aid system. In ensuring sustainability in development projects the study (Hossain 1998b) primarily framed three influential factors and found that sustainability of NGO-led development projects largely dependent on: (a.) Environment in target country, (b.) Donors' commitment to the project, and (c.) Operating NGOs managerial capacity to implement the project.

The study found that the **target country environment** is not necessarily hostile to the professional development of NGOs, rather the government policies in Bangladesh and Nepal are quite supportive to the sector. Government tries to control NGO activities, such control also exists elsewhere in the world. However, control should not cause suffering for NGOs. There are problems with the control – what might not necessarily connected to the hostile attitude of the governments towards NGOs and their development approach. Those problems might be more connected to the power, politics and poverty, e.g. corruption, prejudice, unconsciousness, illiteracy, etc. Some internal and external elite also benefits from these problems. Probably, not only NGO sector, also other institutions i.e. private and public sectors are also equally facing these problems. Democratic exercise in national politics is quite new in both countries—there exists oligarchy to different extent, that might create problems for NGOs to function. In Nepal, development NGOs are quite new, thus would take time for the state structures to respond to this new approach in development. After the rise and fall of NGO-government relation in past governments in both countries have accepted NGOs as a development partner – future remains to be seen.

Donors' commitment is the factor what has strengthened the growth of NGOs in developing countries and their flexibility in commitment, also risking for the sustainability of this sector. Donor aid to NGOs is not any separate factor from the global response of poverty, aid, market and civil society. Probably, donors ideological commitment is more important than professional commitment e.g. commitment for profit, hidden agenda, etc. Still, certain degree of uncertainty is felt among the Southern NGOs about the donors' commitment – at least in Bangladesh and Nepal that is the case.

The **management capacity of NGOs** in both countries is very weak. There does not even exist any major initiative by the donors or by the governments to improve the capacity of NGOs. Some NGOs are doing well in their project management, some are not managing well at all – like some other government or private agencies. There is a big risk to ensure sustainability without building basic understanding on project management. Without proper management of NGO-led development projects the NGO sector is also about to lose its believed comparative advantage in development aid practise — as mentioned earlier that their comparative advantage is highly questioned in aid literature. Giving knowledge of project management to the NGO personnel could be an important step and strategic choice for the governments, donors, and NGOs in ensuring sustainability of their projects. At least providing primary knowledge on the factors of strategic management i.e. Projects environment, strategy, structure and process (Paul 1986) could be a good tool for future development and sustainability of NGOs.

REFERENCES

Abed, F. H. et al (1984): *NGO Efforts and Planning. Development as an Experimental Process*, paper presented at a seminar on Focus of 50 Million: Poverty in Bangladesh, organised by ADAB, Dhaka. 1984

Aminuzzaman, Salahuddin & Begum, Afroza (2000): NGOs and the institutional framework of poverty alleviation: Experiences and lessons from Bangladesh. In: Hossain, Farhad & Ulvila, Marko & Newaz, Ware (Eds.; 2000): *Learning NGOs and the Dynamics of Development Partnership*. Dhaka: Ahsania Books. P. 97-127

Aminuzzaman, Salahuddin (1994) *GOB-NGO Interface. An Institutional Analysis*. Dhaka: Department of Public Administration, University of Dhaka

Aminuzzaman, Salahuddin (1998): NGOs and the grassroot base local government in Bangladesh: A study of their institutional interactions. In: Hossain, Farhad & Myllylä, Susanna (Eds.: 1998): *NGOs Under Challenge: Dynamics and Drawbacks in Development*. Helsinki: Ministry for Foreign Affairs of Finland, Department for International Development Co-operation. P. 84-104

Anheier, Helmut K. & Seibel, Wolfgang (Eds.: 1990): *The Third Sector. Comparative Studies of Nonprofit Organizations*. Berlin: Walter de Gruyter

Asian Development Bank (1994): *Women in Development: Issues, Challenges and Strategies in Asia and the Pacific*. Manila: Asian Development Bank.

Bista, Dor Bahadur (1994): *Fatalism and Development. Nepal's Struggle for Modernization*. Calcutta: Orient Longman

Chaudhary, Churna Bahadur (1998): *BASE Nepal* (An unpublished monograph & office record). Tulsipur/Dang: Backward Society Education

Dhakal, Tek Nath & Hossain, Farhad (1999): *The Fate of Ghewa Tamang and the Mercy of Non-Governmental Organisations: The Impact & Relevance of Development Initiatives in Nepal*. (Unpublished draft) Working Document. NGOs in Development Research Project. Tampere, Finland: University of Tampere, Department of Administrative Science, & Kathmandu, Nepal: Tribhuvan University, Central Department of Public

Administration

Fowler, Alan (1992): *Building Partnerships between Northern and Southern Development NGOs.* Issues for the Nineties. Development, No. 1, p. 16-23

Hossain, Farhad & Dhakal, Tek Nath (1999): *Public, Private & Non-profits: Institutional Analysis of Hekuli VDC of Dang District in Mid-Western Nepal.* (Unpublished draft) Working Document. NGOs in Development Research Project. Tampere, Finland: University of Tampere, Department of Administrative Science, & Kathmandu, Nepal: Tribhuvan University, Central Department of Public Administration.

Hossain, Farhad & Ulvila, Marko & Khan, Iqbal Ansary (1999): *Evaluation of the Health Programme of the Bangladesh Lutheran Mission - Finnish.* Vantaa, Finland: Finnish Lutheran Overseas Mission and Naogaon, Bangladesh: Bangladesh Lutheran Mission-Finnish

Hossain, Farhad (1998): Development in Nepal: Possibilities through Non-governmental Organisations. In Hossain, Farhad & Myllylä, Susanna (Eds.) (1998): *NGOs Under Challenge. Dynamics and Drawbacks in Development.* Helsinki: Ministry for Foreign affairs of Finland, Department for international development Cooperation. pp.105-125

Hossain, Farhad (1998b): *Administration of development projects by Nordic and local Non-Governmental Organisations: A study of their sustainability in South Asian states of Bangladesh and Nepal.* Licentiate thesis. Tampere: University of Tampere, Department of Administrative Science

Hossain, Farhad (2000): Dynamics or Drawbacks: Current issues in NGO research. In: Hossain, Farhad & Ulvila, Marko & Newaz, Ware (Eds.; 2000): *Learning NGOs and the Dynamics of Development Partnership.* Dhaka: Ahsania Books. P. 65-93

Huda, Khawja Shamsul (1987): The Development of NGOs in Bangladesh. In *ADAB News*, Dhaka. May-June 1987.

Hulme, David (1994): Social Development Research and the Third Sector. NGOs as Users and Subjects of Social Inquiry. In: Booth, David (Ed.: 1994): *Rethinking Social Development. Theory, Research & Practice.* Essex: Longman. P. 251-275

IIRR (93-2501EI) *Management problems in nongovernmental organizations.* Manila: International Institute for Rural Reconstruction

Kalimullah, Nazmul Ahsan (1990): Non-Governmental Organizations in Development. Some Conceptual Issues. *Development Review* (Dhaka), Vol. 2, No. 2, p. 165-175.

Khan, A Z M Obaidullah (1990): *Creative Development- an unfinished saga of human aspirations in South Asia.* Dhaka: University Press Limited

Mälkiä, Matti & Hossain, Farhad (1998): Changing Patterns of Development Co-operation: Conceptualising Non-Governmental Organisations in Development. In Hossain, Farhad & Myllylä, Susanna (Eds.) (1998):

NGOs Under Challenge. Dynamics and Drawbacks in Development. Helsinki: Ministry for Foreign affairs of Finland, Department for international development Cooperation. pp.22-46.

National Planning Commission- NPC Nepal (1997): *The Ninth Plan 1997-2002.* Kathmandu: National Planning Commission, HMG/N

Nepal South Asia Center (1998): *Nepal Human Development Report 1998.* Kathmandu: Nepal South Asia Center

Oakley, Peter & Marsden, David (1990): *Approaches to Participation in Rural Development.* Geneva: International Labour Office.

OECD (1989): *Sustainability in Development Programmes: A Compendium of Evaluation Experience. Selected Issues in Aid Evaluation - 1.* Paris: OECD

Paul, Samuel (1986): *Strategic Management of Development Programmes.* Geneva: International Labour Office (ILO)

Quibria, M. G. (ed.) (1994): *Rural Poverty in Developing Asia. Volume 1.* Manila: Asian Development Bank.

Riddel, Roger C. & Bebbington, Anthony & Peck, Lennart (1995): *Promoting Development by Proxy - The Development Impact of Government Support to Swedish NGOs.* London: Overseas Development Institute.

Siddiqui, Kamal (ed.) (1992): *Local Government in South Asia- A Comparative Study.* Dhaka: University Press Limited.

Tvedt, Terje (1995): *Non-governmental Organizations as Channel in Development Assistance.* The Norwegian System. Oslo: Royal Ministry of Foreign Affairs.

Tvedt, Terje (1997): *Development NGOs - actors in a new international social system.* Bergen: A draft paper presented at the conference "Non-Governmental Organisations in aid. A reappraisal of 35 years of NGO assistance". 3-5 November 1997.

Tvedt, Terje (1998): NGOs' Role at 'The End of History': Norwegian Policy and the New Paradigm. In: Hossain, Farhad & Myllylä, Susanna (Eds.: 1998): *NGOs Under Challenge: Dynamics and Drawbacks in Development.* Helsinki: Ministry for Foreign Affairs of Finland, Department for International Development Co-operation. P. 60-83

Ulvila, Marko & Saifullah, A. K. M. & Hossain, Farhad (2000): *Institutional analysis of Biswhanathpur village (Netrokona, Bangladesh) with emphasis on non-governmental organisations.* Working document. NGOs in Development Research Project. Tampere: University of Tampere, Department of Administrative Science

UNDP (1998): *Human Development Report 1998.* New York: UNDP, Oxford University Press

United Nations (1995) *Press Release SOC/4365,* March 13. Copenhagen: UN World Summit for Social Development

University of Dhaka (1994): *Study on the Role of NGOs and Their Institutional*

Interactions with the Local Government in Bangladesh. Dhaka: Department of Public Administration

Interviews

Ahmed, Salehuddin, Director General, NGO Affairs Bureau, Prime Minister's Office, Dhaka. Interviewed in Dhaka on 15.4.1996 by Farhad Hossain.

Chaudhari, Hallu Prasad, Education Programme Co-ordinator, Backward Education Society, Dang. Interviewed in Tulsipur, Dang on 19.5.1999 and [11.7.1999] by Tek Nath Dhakal and [Farhad Hossain]

Pokharel, Tika Prasad, Member Secretary, Social Welfare Council (SWC), Nepal. Interviewed in Kathmandu on 10.8.1999 by Farhad Hossain and Tek Nath Dhakal

Rokeya, Begum, Project Director, Sabalamby Unnayan Samity, Netrokona. Interviewed in Netrokona on 6.4.1996 by Farhad Hossain.

4. CONCEPTUALISING DEVELOPMENT ENCOUNTERS: THE CASE OF THE FINNS IN NEPAL

Mari Poikolainen

INTRODUCTION

In this article, I address the concept of field in cultural analysis and its possible implications in analysing NGOs from an anthropological point of view. The concept of field is treated as a uncritically applied stance of anthropological endeavour to understand other cultures, i.e., those in the South as the Other vs. the Self at home in the North. After a more general and theoretical discussion I aim at demonstrating these issues in two NGO settings: Finnish missionaries and volunteers in Nepal[3] as studied by a Finnish anthropologists.

CONCEPTIONS OF THE FIELD IN NGO CONTEXTS

Despite a self-reflective turn in anthropology since 1980´s Akhil Gupta and James Ferguson argue that there has not been much critical reflection on the field and fieldwork, which still hold a central role in anthropology. They are embedded in implicit presumptions, that guide the anthropological research paradigm since Bronislaw Malinowski set the standards in the first half of this century. Fieldwork and participant observation are still held for the founding stones of the discipline that make it distinct from other academic disciplines. (Gupta & Ferguson 1997: 2, 7.) Here I take up a few of such implicit norms, participant observation, geographically restricted unit of study, and requirement for distance, and relate them to studying NGOs. I also discuss change in research topics towards modern phenomena such as NGOs and new potential ways of making anthropology.

In symbolic, constructivist and discourse based research, which makes a strong vein in current anthropology along with a more empirically oriented scientific anthropology (Hackenberg 1999: 212-213.) participant observation is rather problematic. "Being there" in the field matters, in my view, but merely as an aide in contextualising and understanding textual worlds produced in the interviews, not as much as a means of proving what was said as "of the reality". What does field stand for in the context of a discourse oriented study of the Finnish missionaries and volunteers in development co-operation in Nepal? Does it comprise studying their family and friends, work places and involvement in

---

[3] This discussion is based on an ongoing research titled "Cultures in Development Co-operation: The Finns in Nepal" which includes also development consultants as a third case of Finns in Nepal. The work was initiated in 1998 and fieldwork was conducted in Finland and in Nepal in 1999.

NGOs or leisure in Nepal (a geographically distant country from Finland)? They might seem the most obvious places to focus on in a more scientifically oriented anthropology. But in Nepal as well as in Finland the Finns do not form a bounded community that could be researched through participant observation. They lead their individual or family lives in various locations in Nepal depending on the work that they are assigned to do for the receiving NGO. Some of them keep in touch with other Finns, some do it less. Hence, participant observation (more appropriately applied to bounded units of study), does not provide comprehensive means to study the Finns in Nepal either. Here interviews with the involved Finns as the main source of material (eventually understood as constructed texts) combined with participation in some of the activities of the Finns is a way of trespassing the limits of participant observation.

Distinction to "home" and "the field" creates hierarchy of purity of field sites in anthropology. Some field sites, still most often those that are far away and least integrated to the industrial society are regarded as more authentic than those that are close, industrial and urban. Anthropologist Mary Des Chene notes that however intense the participation, eventually the fieldworker is left with an outsider's view of a community. Tendency to concentrate on the present is inevitable (particularly in communities with no written language) due to lacking language skills and other restrictions of being an outsider. (Des Chene 1997: 68.) Des Chene argues that the requirement for distance has naturalised "the field":

> Just as 'the Other' is a designation that strips people of cultural and historical particularity, 'the Field' strips places of their specificity; as the object and ground of anthropological practice, both 'the Other' and 'the Field' become ahistoricized conceptual entities, transformed by the ethnographic gaze. (Des Chene 1997: 70.)

Following Des Chene's critical notion of the homogenised and present-oriented field, in the context of the Finns involved in NGO activities in Nepal the field can be seen as multiple fields. The field is not merely either geographically (near or far) or socially bounded unit accessible through participant observation but a series of time-bound events ("real" or textually constructed) in search of discourses. In practical terms, the field seems to consist of communication with the Finns while interviewing them. But it can be seen to include also the constructed mental or textual realities that the Finns create in their talk of working in NGOs in Nepal. Hence, the field is not ahistorical, but tied to the stories of the past, present and future.

Yet another temporal aspect of the field is that the Finns live in Nepal only temporarily. Most of them eventually move on back to Finland or another country. Their time in Nepal is tied to contract terms and hence is temporary which gives a special flavour to their stay as a whole and to the way they talk about it. Often the receiving NGOs employ other Finnish expatriates after they leave. From the point of view of the NGO there is continuity in the Finnish presence but not from that of an individual Finn. However, the individual Finns are affected by the organisational continuity and that is conveyed in the talk of the Finns as well. Interviews prove useful from this perspective as well.

Kath Weston deconstructs questions of participation, distance and proximity in the light of native anthropology which she claims to have been marginalised in the periphery of mainstream anthropology. (Weston 1997: 163, 179.) According to Weston native anthropologists are seen as part of their group of origin and as a compound of various identity categories attached to it. Naturalisation creates a virtual anthropologist and Native Ethnographer, who is an imaginary hybrid destined to utilise certain identity categories (such as ethnicity, race, nation state). Native anthropologist's work is always a little removed from "the real anthropology". (Weston 1997: 163, 170, 178.)

> Excised and tokenized, the virtual anthropologist inherits much of the loneliness associated with the outsider-within position, but little of its fixity. Her problems do not stem from being a dyke out of (her) place in academe, but from those seemingly unpredictable shifts from Native to Ethnographer and back again. (Weston 1997: 178.)

In anthropology the nativisation is related to constructing "the Other" at distance as distinct from "the Self" and home. The gradual change in perceiving "home" (the Self) and "the field" (the Other) in anthropology is related partially to the dismantling of colonialism. Since the Western anthropologists had connection to and had been using the facilities provided by colonial powers, they were seen as less welcome visitors in the newly independent countries and former colonies. The field could be or even had to be imagined and constructed ethnographically at home in the West or at home elsewhere. Implicit appreciation for distance and fieldwork as *rite de passage* for anthropologists as living in the communities they investigate had and has to be reconsidered. (see, e.g., Hannerz 1996.)

In the context of studying the Finns and their involvement in development NGOs in Nepal, being a Finn and a researcher makes my position in Weston's terms unpredictable. The categories of the Other and the Self are mixed to some extent; the Other being the Finns in Nepal and the Self similarly being the Finns in Nepal. Only particular situations reveal whether it is the position of the Other (e.g., researcher in interviews and participant observer in NGO settings) or that of the Self (a Finn among other Finns in Nepal) that is being emphasised. Acknowledging the situationality of these positions dismantles the ahistorical dimension of both "the field" and "the Other" and makes the analysis transparent as to the entitlements of each party.

Several new approaches for anthropological field practise have been suggested. Solutions for studying transitory phenomena, such as migratory work, are sought after in various kinds of notions of non-local fieldwork (e.g., Marcus 1996). Fieldwork integrating several methods and multi-locale in nature responds better to the challenges brought by new phenomena characterised by mobility (of people and of goods) and by fusion of local and global elements. A potentially applicable notion of the field for studying NGOs is suggested by Gupta & Ferguson. They pay attention to the field not as a geographical place but as multiple locations and propose to pay attention to location instead of the local. They coin the concept *location-work* as a continuous and constructive alternative for the conventional field and fieldwork in anthropology. (Gupta & Ferguson 1997: 5.)

> ...it seems most useful to us to attempt to redefine the fieldwork "trademark" not with a time-honored commitment to the *local* but with an attentiveness to social, cultural and political *location* and a willingness to work self-consciously at shifting or realigning our own location while building epistemological and political links with other locations. (Gupta & Ferguson 1997: 5.)

The distinction to social, cultural and political location of field and fieldwork captures the situational nature of the field also in connection to the Finns in development NGOs in Nepal better than the conventional fixed notion of the local field. Hence, the field is not about being in a place, it is about communication, knowledge and power, i.e., social, cultural and political location. It involves continuous reflection of meaning and relations of locations of the researched and the researcher. If the field is not limited to geographical terms (local) but is seen in a broader sense as cultural, social and political location, non-local source materials that construct location are available to anthropological investigation. For instance, interviews with the Finns can be seen as non-local source material. They construct location through interaction and communication.

Similarly, Des Chene emphasise the importance of historical material and perspective in anthropology, that extend the synchronic perspective of field as local. Des Chene conceives historical material as *historically situated field* and in relation to conventional field attached to the local: the field is not necessarily a place at all but rather a historical era or series of events that take the researcher to several locations. (Des Chene 1997: 76-81.) Hence, any piece of anthropological research utilising archives or even more temporary material such as organisational news letters of NGOs the notion of historically situated field becomes applicaple..

As briefly mentioned above, "the field" as an anthropological construction is undergoing change due to challenges new transitory and mobile phenomena of the present, that are by and by being incorporated into mainstream anthropology, carry with them (Malkki 1997: 86.). Migration, refugees, work abroad, and the Internet, to name but a few, require anthropology to redefine its scope and practices. Liisa Malkki (echoing Benedict Anderson's concept of imagined community[4]), talks about *accidental communities of memory* that are born after certain local and temporal events are not existing any more. The fieldworker of such events cannot go back to the time and place of the already dissolved events. There has to be other ways of constructing the space of the events. The events can be reconstructed from several sources, e.g., written and oral accounts. Here as well, the field is not local but rather an accidental community of memory which live and is constructed in the stories of those people who had been involved in the events. (Malkki 1995) NGO settings of the Finns in Nepal make a vivid example of such transitory phenomena. In concrete terms, the Finns work for the receiving NGOs for some time (from a few months to several years) but eventually most of them leave for other assignments. "The NGO space of events" can be still constructed through memories of those involved, e.g., through interviews with both the Finns still in Nepal and the Finns already back in Finland. In the interviews the memories are created through textual means and can be, hence, studied as discourses.

Coming gradually to the point, all of these notions of non-local field seem to give validity to studying NGOs through anthropological means as well, despite them being modern and transitory (to the people involved) as opposed to distant and stable. NGOs both "at home" and elsewhere have similar features from the methodological point of view. These features can be captured through a mixture of methods varying from interviews to archives and news letters. The common ground of them all is that they provide means to the textual construction of NGO as sites of communication, knowledge, and power, that is perhaps still not addressed adequately. William Fisher even argues that NGO discourse tends to sustain antipolitics referring to the obscuring of power-structured relationships in everyday life (Fisher 1997: 446.). By dismantling the homogenising notions of the field supports a more diversified picture of NGOs.

In the above discussion I have come to describe the central aspects of the field in the context of the Finnish missionaries and volunteers in development NGOs in Nepal. I lean on ideas of location-work, historically situated field, and accidental communities of memory brought up by Gupta & Ferguson, Des Chene and Malkki in determining the field and its meaning. Their practical implications are demonstrated in the next section of the article together with issues concerning culture and NGOs in development.

POSITIONING OF AND IN DEVELOPMENT NGOS

When analysing the discourse of development Arturo Escobar talks about the institutionalised field of development discourse "from which discourses are produced, recorded, stabilised, modified, and put into circulation" (Escobar 1995,

---

[4] "...all communities beyond the size of a closed village are abstractly imagined by their members, but the style of imagining differs." (Eriksen 1993: 91, referring to Anderson.)

39-47). Since the 1940's institutionalisation of development took place at all levels, from international to local levels, including NGOs. Escobar maintains that together with professionalisation it created particular forms of power and means of relating to each other. It is within this framework, that people operating in the field of development are bound to. Therefore, NGOs are essentially part of the wider development discourse; they have their constantly renegotiated role in the production and distribution of knowledge and power. (Escobar 1995, 39-47; see also Crush 1995 and Cowen & Shenton 1996). Moreover, the concept of equity is closely related to power. Walter Van Beek maitains that: "The realisation that all have different stakes in development is crucial, as is the fact that these stakes though all bear their own legitimacy, operate from different positions of power." (van Beek 1995, 279)

A UNESCO publication *The Cultural Dimension of Development* from 1995 maintains that:

> "The work of NGOs, very different as it is from that of the large bilateral and multilateral co-operation agencies, is of considerable value primarily in terms of cultural sensitivity and the quality of the results achieved." (Almeida-Klein 1995, 77)

This view frequently held for NGOs stating that their grass-root orientation and catalyst role are their greatest advantages compared to other agents in development, is put into a larger picture by situating them in Escobar's manner in wider discourse. Thierry Verhelst also represents this commonly shared position of putting high value on NGOs in general (Verhelst 1990). He is, to put it in Jan Nederveen Pieterse's terms, "along with much of the grassroots oriented alternative development approach, homogenizing the subaltern, at other times ascribing a romantic role to grassroots intellectuals". (Neederveen Pieterse 1995, 39) In a similar fashion, van Beek raises the question of communication and information in development. He points out that national or regional governments, or NGOs for that matter, are not to be entitled to define the problems and wishes of host-populations. They are, in fact, constituting "a third party with its own culture and priorities". In van Beek's view: "The fact that they are allowed to think of themselves as the interpreters only increases misunderstanding." (van Beek 1995, 278.) By viewing NGOs as part of the current development discourse, as institutionalised agents in it, it is possible to open up ways to analyse their role as part of the production of power relations and as agents in translocal negotiation of strategic boundaries. In the next, I attempt to juxtapose the preceding discussion of the field (and culture) with that of the role of NGOs in the context of the Finnish missionaries and volunteers in development co-operation in Nepal.

As mentioned previously, besides interviews with the Finns, the field includes selected publications such as training material and newsletters published by the involved NGOs as well as circular letters sent by missionaries to their home parishes in Finland. Des Chene notes that:

> Moving around (or not) as necessary and seeking traces of the past are two of many ways we might be able to achieve a less extractive kind of research, to study villages, (towns, neighborhoods...) not just study *in* them, while still (or rather thereby) illuminating larger patterns and processes (or, as the current jargon has it, global flows)." (Des Chene 1997, 79)

I attempt to capture traces of commonalties and differences in the Finnish talk on their experiences in Nepal as well as traces of the (rather recent) past in organisational documents. The field is not restricted locally (to a place) but includes several temporal and spatial as well as also political, cultural and social locations. I aim at substantiating this with some examples. It need to be stressed that this is a rather exploratory enterprise and may contain interpretations beyond the scope of the original concept of location-work. In my view, location-work can be fruitfully related to Nederveen Piederse's views of the wholeness of culture as situationally relevant, strategic sets of improvisations. Location-work and strategic improvisation emphasise the relevance of situational, time-bound and actor-oriented nature of culture (Nederveen Piederse 1995, 43.). They can be used in research to avoid looking for structural and coherent entities (to prove grand theories) and instead can be used to highlight significant issues as a process. The situationality makes issues significant not any fixed categories outside them such as nationality, gender, attachment to an NGO etc. In the next, I illuminate this stance by discussing the significance of nation state, development co-operation and NGOs, and leisure as shifting locations of meaning.

It is easy to think of culture as a territorial category, local or national. But as mentioned earlier culture can be seen as a historically situated strategic choice and reaction to current conditions, whereby it is neither territorial nor structural (fixed categories), but can be said to be translocal. By viewing culture as translocal is an open conception. In that case, the wholeness of cultures consists in their being "situationally relevant, strategic sets of improvisations" (Nederveen Pieterse 1995, 43.). For the Finns in Nepal, nation state (Finnish or Nepalese) may in some cases, construct cultural location (symbols and menings), and in other cases political location (power relations). It is not a fixed category with always the same features. Neither Finland, nor Nepal is necessarily significant as a geographical entity, their significance is, on one hand, related to power hierarchy and political location-work they are part of. The meaning of nation states arises in their ability to manipulate and use power recognisable even in everyday situations. Bilateral development co-operation entails mutually accepted official agreements on the distribution of resources which translate to power and authority. This setting influences the relations of the citizens of these countries in everyday activities, e. g., there are those people, who have power to decide upon economic matters and those who manipulate this power.

Moreover, in many cases, the Westerners tend to stand for power and money in the eyes of non-Westerners even if they were volunteers or missionaries with no or little pay. They say they feel to become, therefore, often targets of manipulation. In a very concrete way, this is evident particularly in tourist areas in Nepal, where Westerners, including the expatriate Finns, are not left with any doubt that they could share some of her wealth against services or goods. This kind of homogenisation can be particularly frustrating for the Finns (or any Westerner) living in Nepal for years or even decades.

> R: But in a way, I mean, it has been a topic in so many discussions how you gain such a bad mood when you come to Thamel (touristic central Kathmandu). When you should should shop something, for example souvenirs, should buy whatever whenever, and should come to Thamel. So I mean, you feel so bad or it frustrates immensely that you are held for a toursit all the time. Someone tries to sell you something all the time and the like. (A Finnish volunteer in Nepal)

Conversely, the Nepalese can be understood by the Finnish as holding things to themselves as a form of power practice. For instance, at work the authority and power is not tied to being an expert in a manner that it would be in Finland, which makes it harder to participate on an equal (as understood by the Finns) basis. It is not tied to being a Westerner in the sense of representing a donor either which can be a bit confusing, since that is in some ways expected.

> R: That there are terribly, I mean, sort of top-down kind of leadership. And sometimes it is an awful shock to realise that I am so low in the hierarchy.

> Q: Even if you are, ee, it does not affect you that you are a Westerner, so that it does not make you rise in the hierarchy...?

> R: No, it doesn't, but because of the fact that I did not have, I mean, I have authority based on expertise. So authority tied to expertise does not necessarily make a person rise in the hierarchy over here. That for example I mean in practice that many sort of policies or pla- plans or the like. They are not told to you. About money you have to always go and try to find out yourself.

> Q: Yeah.

> R: Even if you come from the side of the donor, so to speak. (A Finnish missionary in Nepal)

This shows that being a Finn has different implications depending on the situations, e.g., at work. The background in a Finnish nation state as a wealthy Western donor affects the positioning of both the Finns and of the Nepalis. Despite of it being linked to (by themselves and by others) money and power it is not always the case that the Finns have either of them. In some cases, the nation state position makes a meaningful situating strategy, but not always.

Cultural location work in relation to nation state can be viewed as a process of making distinctions. First, a few words of the concept of culture. Nederveen Pieterse calls for a critical view on romanticising views on local culture as the last frontier of cultural authenticity. He perceives it dangerous to homogenise local communities as local cultures reminiscent of classical sociologists' terminology of *Gemeinschaft* or *organic solidarity* (see also Banuri 1995, 40). The local does not exist as such, but is a strategy "in construction and negotiation of external boundaries". It is as culture, a multiply authored invention. (Nederveen Pieterse 1995, 36.) The Finns living in Nepal make distinctions at times on the basis of nationality. Occasionally, Finland appears to be a target of identification or at least to give meaning and orientation of experiences and knowledge. In other occasions links are stressed to Nepal, particularly in discussions with other Finns in Finland. There even seem to appear to a certain extend a competitive spirit among the expatriates over who has valid authority to say something of the country. Additionally, during the course of a single conversation belonging and boundary building terms such as "we" and "they" may refer to a variety of people: the other Finns, the Nepalese, the Christians, the Lutherans[5], or the other foreigners. "We" and "they" stand for different meanings (and several identity categories) depending on the context. (Eriksen 1993) The nation state categories are not necessarily any more determining than the other categories. Overall, nation state constructs both political (power and authority) and cultural (making distinctions) location among other elements in the overall process of location-work.

Further implications of location-work can be detected in the NGO affiliations of missionaries and volunteers. From the point of view of activities the Finns are occupied in development co-operation in Nepal. Development work contains the implicit notion of change. The Finnish missionaries and volunteers are attached to NGOs with different notions of what change and development entail as well as with different notions of knowledge and power relations. Commonalties within an organisation lie in how development is believed to be best nurtured. NGOs can be seen to construct political location, a particular and distinct stance towards power and knowledge linkages of development co-operation.

Apart from the organisational documents and mission statements of each NGO political location can be identified in the talk of missionaries and volunteers. The Finnish missionaries, who I met, emphasise the actual development work over any religious ambitions but still they say they would preferably work for a missionary NGO rather than any NGO.

> Q: Yeah, ee, could you say that you have experienced a call to become a missionary or is it more like something....

---

[5] Evangelical Lutheran Christianity is the dominant religious denomination in Finland.

R: Yes, yeah, I mean, when I was younger I had that kind of feel what it might be, but now after 1993 I have had a clear missionary call and the call has come.

Q: Yeah, yeah.

R: So that it has to do with such a process of spiritual life where I have experienced that God has clearly called me. (A Finnish missionary in Nepal)

The development work of missionaries involves striving for (material) change. In their leisure they are free to do what they want, and hence, also engage in dialogue with the local people on spiritual issues ("spiritual" change). The Finnish volunteers who are attached to local child rights and environmental NGOs come to Nepal with the idea of internationalisation through personal experiences in mind. They are even trained not to believe to be able to change much, if anything in a few months that they usually stay in Nepal. The emphasis is on mutual respectful contact not on any real (material) change.

In the talk of missionaries and volunteers it is possible to identify some features of the social location-work such as identification with the social community NGOs create. Their background organisations form political location in relation to other actors of development co-operation. The missionary NGO of missionaries and the child rights and environmental NGOs of volunteers do not automatically form communities because people in one organisation do not necessarily even work geographically near each other or have direct contacts to one other. The work communities of the Finns are multinational with mixed teams of Finnish, other international and Nepalese workers together. Many Finns avoid making generalisations when asked to describe their co-operation with Nepalese people at work and leisure in Nepal. They rather emphasise the diversity and uniqueness of situations.

R: Yea, if you think that at work with international team, one might easily think that the Westerners understand each other easier. But the fact that we come from different backgrounds and come from different Western countries, so, it is a momentum as such. So that the assumption that it is easier to get along with the Westerners than with the Nepalis is erroneous. I mean, such a presumption in my case. In my view, it is not that that that, it is not... it is more influenced by the status and personality than the fact which country you come from. (A Finnish missionary in Nepal)

Hence, within an NGO the nationality of its members does not necessarily draw people together even if working with people from one country may be sometimes easier than with people from another country. The NGO work community of missionaries at project level may, however, construct social location in form of tasks connecting people socially to each other, or at times even, in form of geographical closeness (bounded unit).

For volunteers the work community does not necessarily play any major role, since they are often only loosely integrated to the organisation of the receiving NGO, e.g., due to lacking skills in Nepali language and the shortness of their stay. Instead of social location the NGO work community may create political location in terms of decision-making, e.g., in questions of who has the power to decide over the use of resources and over participation in various tasks.

The cultural location-work in NGO contexts can be understood to involve making distinctions to other people based on values and symbols. At work the Finns are tied to the official bilateral agreements of the nations as well as organisations. They reflect to certain degree their NGO background and policies. In leisure they are freer to express their personal values and ambitions, and it can be taken, hence, particularly as a site for cultural location work. For volunteers, who are not and whose work is not as integrated to the rest of the work community, the leisure tends to become central. Many volunteers live in local families and have, thus, opportunity to learn of the everyday life of the local family. Issues such as when to wake up, when and how to have meals, when to come home in the evenings are constantly being negotiated. Some volunteers tend to identify as the most notable difference to their life in Finland the "excess" time at long dark evenings, that they normally would use for, e.g., hobbies, friends or watching television. In Nepal that time appears like a rather empty gap between sleep and daily activities.

Overall, during their relatively short stay in Nepal (about 2-8 months) volunteers are in several processes of cultural location-work. Apart from the local family, there is another point of reference and aspect of positioning themselves in Nepal: tourists.

Q: Yea. Is it exactly that you in a way experience that you are not a tourist.

R: Yeah.

Q: Yeah.

R: About that, there was once some discussion with X (another Finnish volunteer) how one feels so bad coming to Thamel (touristic central Kathmandu), but then he realised that he should take it so that he actually is a tourist. He just is a tourist and in that way he feels better going to Thamel.

Q: Have you tried out that too?

R: I don't, I don't want to think that I am a tourist.

Q: Not at any stage?

R: Well, of course you tend to do certain touristic things occasionally, and then I only lough that now I am a proper tourist. But generally speaking I feel that in some ways I am different to these basic tourists who wander around in Thamel. (A Finnish volunteer in Nepal, 1999.)

Volunteers tend to contemplate their relations to the tourists in one way or another which hints that the issue signifies something to them. Some volunteers acknowledge that they are actually tourists, others want to stay apart and belong clearer to the category of volunteers. Volunteers in the latter sense are regarded as having "a more valued" position in the hierarchy relating various groups of foreigners in Nepal to one another.

For a missionary working in Nepal for years the leisure plays a different role for several reasons. It is time for themselves and their families who usually accompany them in Nepal. It stands for time off from demanding work, which occupies more time in Nepal with its six-day week than in Finland with five-day week. In this sense, it is as if being off service. More significantly, it also stands for time for dialogue which is an essential part of being a missionary. In this sense, it is about being in service of the gospel. Before actually taking on a job they and their families have undergone an extensive period of language and cultural training of about eighteen months. They are, therefore, able to communicate and potentially can create personal relationships and dialogue with local people better than what volunteers can. Missionaries regret that it is relatively difficult to establish genuine and equal dialogue with the local people. They feel that they tend to represent prestige (e.g., through education), wealth (despite their relatively low wages compared with their home countries) and power unobtainable for most local people, which prevents equal relationships. On some occasions these hindrances to dialogue can be set aside:

> R: ..... I think that a good example of, even in all this inequality, that there can be even here. So I think that there are are some certain people who, X a Nepalese doctor, who you feel that you are the same same, I mean it is very easy to talk about anything with him. Well, he is, I mean, an educated person. And then there is this guy from the parish who I regularly meet and who is not educated, but who is really like, with him I experience the same that we are really equal. But then about this equality issue I remember once a poor family invited us for a meal. And then there were the children of the family that were hungry. And of course they had prepared a chicken, cut the head and they give us this delicious chicken. And somehow I did not, I was not going to, the children needed the chicken more than we did. Z (wife) said that now you eat it and enjoy it. And I think that that was sort of reciprocal.... and and it was good, that meal. So that if someone gives you something, someone who you have maybe...given something, so it is now your chance to be the receiver.... But I mean this receiving and giving, and even learning to receive things and. That is where equality becomes reality in some ways. (A Finnish missionary in Nepal.)

Missionaries have settled routines for time off including church activities, school gatherings, and get-togethers with friends (from church, work, and the neighbourhood). An important aspect of leisure for both volunteers and missionaries is that it enables them to withdraw to solitude, that they regularly miss in Nepal. It is a distinct way of gathering strength, that makes them feel different from other people and is referred to as being an integral part of being a

Finn. In short, leisure entails several processes of cultural location work. Some are similar to missionaries and volunteers, others different.

The concept of location-work can be fruitfully related to the concept of accidental community of memory coined by Malkki, which create the actual events (political, cultural and social contexts) textually even after the actual settings have disappeared. In actual terms, the Finns do not form a community in Nepal or may only vaguely know of each other. The continuity and community, if they are accepted to be fundamental characteristics of culture, in studying the Finns in Nepal can be reached through the concept of accidental communities of memory. Such communities are not locally defined: the focus lies on textual means, such as memories and stories told in the interviews, utilised by people to situate themselves, to make distinctions and to create "the Other", be that Other, e.g., the Nepalese or the other Finns from another background (missionaries for volunteers and vice versa).

CONCLUSIONS

In the previous paragraphs I aimed at illuminating the significance of nation state, development co-operation and NGOs as well as leisure as shifting locations of meaning in the context of the Finns development co-operation in Nepal. I believe that the meanings are bound to each particular situation in time and space. In the Finnish discourses on development co-operation in Nepal I looked rather more generally into issues of situating and locating oneself. I took location-work to illuminate some aspects of the hybrid nature of existence of expatriates in Nepal. The Finns draw from many sources for the meaning of their existence which is not possible to reduce to any separate identity categories as such. They constantly work at their location.

Paul Willis, a prominent figure in British cultural studies, claims that anthropology, in all its empiricism (fieldwork) does not still pay attention to politico-economic and historical factors but rather concentrates on micro level issues at the cost of theoretical analysis (Willis 1997, 184.). In anthropology, we do empirical fieldwork and still often manage to avoid any practical implications later in the analysis. We do neither applied nor really theoretical research. In Nepal I learnt anew that applied anthropology is in great demand in development projects (for various reasons). In the West we tend to get overexcited about theoretical formulations and leave practical applications aside. In this vein, studying discourses may not appear particularly meaningful either in the context of development co-operation for the reason of it being purely academic. I started, therefore, feeling uncomfortable of conducting research that bears little direct practical relevance. I was, however, convinced that by doing sort of "native anthropology" as a native Finn investigating the other native Finns in Nepal, I could shed light on some cultural conceptions prevailing in development co-operation, from the point of view of the North (in this first phase of the research project), the role of which is ever so frequently neglected in research on development. The reasons for failures of development lie and have to be detected in all ends of the process.

REFERENCES

Almeida-Klein, Susanne (ed.) 1995: *The cultural dimension of development : towards a practical approach*. 1995. Culture and development series. Paris: UNESCO

Banuri, Tariq 1990: Modernization and its Discontents: A Cultural Perspective on the Theories of Development. In Marglin, Apfel & Marglin Stephen 1990: *Dominating Knowledge. Development, Culture and Resistance*. Oxford: Claredon Press.

van Beek, Walter E.A. 1995: Culture and Development: Problems and Recommendations. In De Ruijter, A. & Van Vucht Tijssen, L. (eds): *Cultural Dynamics in Development Process*. Paris and Den Hague: UNESCO Publishing/Netherlands Commission for UNESCO.

Cowen, M. and Shenton, R.W. 1996: *Doctrines of development*. London: Routledge.

Crush, Jonathan (ed.) 1995: *Power of Development*. London and New York: Routledge.

Des Chene, Mary 1997: Locating the Past. In Gupta, Akhil & Ferguson, James (eds.): *Anthropological Locations. Boundaries and Grounds of a Field Science*. Berkeley, Los Angeles, London: University of California Press. 66-85.

Eriksen, Thomas Hylland 1993, *Ethnicity and Nationalism. Anthropological Perspectives*. London: Pluto Press.

Escobar, Arturo 1995: *Encountering Development. The Making and Unmaking of the Third World*. Princeton, New Jersey: Princeton University Press.

Fisher, William 1997: Doing Good? The Politics and Antipolitics of NGO Practices. *Annual Review of Anthropology* 1997. 26: 429-464.

Gupta, Akhil & Ferguson, James 1997: Discipline and Practice: "The Field" as site, Method, and Location in Anthropology. In Gupta, Akhil & Ferguson, James (eds.): *Anthropological Locations. Boundaries and Grounds of a Field Science*. Berkeley, Los Angeles, London: University of California Press.

Hackenberg, Robert A. 1999: Advancing Applied Anthropology: Globalization: Touchstone Policy Concept or Sucked Orange. *Human Organisation*. Vol. 58, No. 2, 1999.

Hannerz, Ulf 1996: *Transnational Connections. Culture, People, Places*. London and New York: Routledge.

Malkki, Liisa 1995: Refugees and Exile: From "Refugee Studies" to the National Order of Things. *Annual Review of Anthropology* 24: 495-523.

Malkki, Liisa 1997: News and Culture: Transitory Phenomena and the Fieldwork Tradition. In Gupta, Akhil & Ferguson, James (eds.): *Anthropological*

Locations. Boundaries and Grounds of a Field Science. Berkeley, Los Angeles, London: University of California Press. 86-101.

Marcus, George E. (1995) Ethnography in/of the world system: The emergence of multi-sited ethnography. *Annual Review of Anthropology* 1995, 24:95-117. Palo Alto, California.

Nederveen Pieterse, Jan (1995) The Cultural Turn in Development: Question of Power. In De Ruijter, A. & Van Vucht Tijssen, L. (eds.) *Cultural Dynamics in Development Process.* Paris and Den Hague: UNESCO Publishing/Netherlands Commission for UNESCO.

Verhelst, Thierry 1993: *Elämän juuret: kulttuuri ja kehitys.* Helsinki: Kehitysyhteistyön palvelukeskus.

Weston, Kath 1997: The Virtual Anthropologist. In Gupta, Akhil & Ferguson, James (eds.): *Anthropological Locations. Boundaries and Grounds of a Field Science.* Berkeley, Los Angeles, London: University of California Press. 163-184.

Willis, Paul 1997: TIES: Theoretically Informed Ethnographic Study. In Nugent, Stephen & Shore, Cris (eds.) *Anthropology and Cultural Studies.* London, Chicago, IL.: Pluto Press. 182-192.

PART II UNDERSTANDING NGO ACTIVITIES IN NEPAL

5. NGOs and Their Functioning in Nepal

Tika Prasad Pokharel

PERCEPTION TOWARDS NGOS

These days people talk much about Non-governmental Social Organizations (NGOs). Their number also is growing day by day in each country irrespective of rich and poor. NGOs have been involved in several aspects of human concern and they are also demonstrating positive results in many ways. But who they are and/or how they have been defined has become a matter of much controversy.

Many people think that all organizations outside the government are non-governmental organizations. To some extent that may be true and it cannot totally be denied. But what about the political parties and their sister organizations? Could they be called NGOs as long as they are not in the government or they do not have chance to form the government ? Likewise, what about the private banks, schools, universities, nursing homes, hospitals, research institutions as well as cooperatives, religious institutions and various other commercial organizations. Could they also be called NGOs ? Similarly, could organizations like Guthies prevelling in certain communities in Nepal since generations, clubs and users' groups opened and operated in various communities and villages be called NGOs.

Probably what our mind and intuition will like to tell about NGOs is something different than the ones expressed above. It could be apprehended and made clear when we examine the fundamental characteristics of the organizations that they must possess to be called themselves NGOs.

CHARACTERISTICS OF NGOS

Any organization to be called NGO must have four basic characteristics. They are:

- Development Oriented
- Non-political
- Democratic in character
- Non-profit making

Primarily the NGOs should be development oriented, weather it is material development or social development or spiritual development. They should try to institute the change in the society. If they are not development oriented and remain inactive from attempting to initiate a change they turn out to be a place for chatting and making fun and their objectives become confusing. Likewise the NGOs should be non-political. They should not involve into active politics and try to gain political power. Nor they should try to be a vehicle for the political parties to gain political power in the hand of any one of such parties. If the NGOs happened to be so they can hardly get unfailing support from each government and survive themselves. But it does not mean that the NGOs should not have inner politics (e.g. NGO politics) within themselves and within their own sector. They need to have this for their own survival and strength and that is acceptable too.

Thirdly NGOs should be democratic in character. They should work strictly within their own constitution and keep the membership open and operational as defined in their constitution. They should also be very much disciplined and work within the established norms. They should not bypass the law of the land and make all their activities transparent, participatory and responsive. In absence of all these, NGOs loose the confidence of the people, government and the donors as well and that will threaten their own survival. In this context everyone should understand that NGOs are survived with the support of the individuals or the government or donor agencies for their fund and they do not have situation like government and/or the private institutions. All NGOs have to start from the scratch and rely on confidence and trust. Last but not the least; the NGOs should not be profit oriented. This means that the profit earned by the NGOs should not go to its board members like the profit goes to their board members and/or shareholders in all other commercial organizations. But it does not mean that NGOs should not seek profit in all cases. It can seek in many cases but it should go to the account of the NGOs and not to its board members as stated above.

Looking from these prospective the political parties and their sister organizations do not fall within the category of NGOs. Their main purpose is to gain or assist to gain the political power. Likewise the commercial organizations such as banks, co-operatives and various other business entities also do not fall within the category of NGOs. They are mainly for commercial purpose and part of their earning goes as dividend to their shareholders. Nor the loose organizations like users groups and clubs etc., who are not institutionalized and are formed for accomplishing a specific task such as construction of a school building or drinking water system and organizing events for making fun for their members, fall within the category of NGOs. NGOs, therefore, could be defined as social organizations democratically established by a group of people of identical interest within the legal framework of the Country and their objectives are not to gain or assist to gain the political power and earn the profit for the benefit of their own members but to keep active for social, economic and spiritual development of the target groups in a legal as well democratic way.

IMPORTANCE OF NGOS

Till 1960s there was a heavy reliance on government all over the world for the purpose of fulfilling the people's need. This led even up to the extent of advocating communism in some parts of the world, which was primarily to bring all the productive assets under the control of the state and, in return, the government was to deliver the entire needs of the people. But gradually it was realized that the government alone was not enough to address all the needs of the people and improve their Socio-economic condition even if the government is good and democratic in character.

The reason is that the governments have many limitations. Among such limitations the important one is their bureaucracy which makes the governments difficult to reach to the people as quickly as it is needed. Nor it can reach to the real problems in a more spontaneous way. Frequent pressures are needed to make it active. Therefore the need of the private sector was started to realize almost in all parts of the world and make this sector more active to supplement the governments in such conditions.

Private sector is guided primarily by profit. If it feels that the profits are possible, it does not mind to go in any place. It can even go to the remotest of the remote and poorest of the poor places. In this context no one has to pressurize it. Hence the private sector has been advocated as a sector to supplement to the government and it has been advocated more extensively particularly, after 1960s.

There is a belief that private sector can reach easily to the places where the government can not reach. But it is not always true. It can reach only when there is an organized market. If the market is unorganized and scattered the private sector is not always willing to be there. In such a situation the notion of creating demand by supply also is not normally true. Hence the places which are too remote and socially and economically backward and where the markets are undeveloped in such places the private sector also does not reach normally as the government does. To fill-in this gaps, therefore, it has been started to advocate the need of the NGOs, which are flexible and can reach easily to the places and people as and when it is needed. They are also cost-effective to a large extent and are participatory. Their programs are relatively sustainable, since they give more attention on generating process and addressing the human issues. NGOs, therefore, have started to get more and more support from all concerns. They have started to gain importance from the developed countries as an effective vehicle to channelize their development supports to the developing countries. They have also started to gain importance as an effective instrument to deliver goods and services in the developing countries where the efficiency on the part of the government as well as the private sector has yet to achieve. NGOs, thus, are growing as a third sector and getting momentum as an effective sector to address the human issues particularly from 1980s.

Although the Social Organizations were functioning in Nepal from generations in different forms in different communities such as Guthies, Dhikuries, Kipat and Bheja[1] etc, the process of emerging Social Organizations in modern from started quite in late. Probably it could be no wrong to mention the name of Gandhi Memorial Charkha Prachar Guthi which was established as a first of such organization in the year 1947 and the main objective of this organization was to involve the deprived communities including the destitute women for spinning and weaving. Gradually the Guthi also took up several other social activities such as education and health care. Later a Paropakar Aushadalaya was established by a group of active people and it was developed as an institute which provided care to the orphans and educational facilities as well as health care services to the week and deprived. Since then Several organizations like Nepal Red Cross Society, Nepal Disabled Association, Leprosy Control Association, Nepal Children organization, TB Control Association etc started to come into existence. But their activities were basically service oriented and they were lacking to coordinate and facilitate centrally.

For the purpose of coordination and facilitation of the Social Organizations and their activities, the need of a central level organization was felt by the then Social Workers and a body was constituted under the chairmanship of Her Majesty the Queen in 1977 by the name Social Service National Coordination Council (SSNCC) . At that time there were altogether 37 Social Organizations associated with SSNCC. The SSNCC, however, was operating outside the main system of the government organization being it chaired by Her Majesty the Queen and it was bound to follow the basic norms of the them political system which used to be called as Panchayat system - a King led partyless system. Such environment did not allow a spontaneous growth of social organizations in Nepal. As a result, till to the March 1990 the total number of local NGOs were altogether 219 and international NGOs were 54 associated with the then SSNCC.

By the year 1989 the political change took place and a multiparty democratic system was restored in the country. As a consequence, Her Majesty the Queen gave away the chairmanship of SSNCC and a new Act known as Social Welfare Act was also brought into existence in 1992. This Act changed the name of Social Service National Coordination Council (SSNCC) to Social Welfare Council (SWC) and the organization was brought within the main

---

[1] Guthies are the organizations functioning in Newar communities to perform social and religious functions limiting within their own members. Dhikuries are informal organizations functioning among Thakali and Gurung communities for the purpose of rotational credit arrangement among their own members. Kipats are the communal land arrangement system operational among Rai, Limbu, Tamang & Jirel communities. Bhejas are the traditional organizations which settle several social issues within the Magar communities.

system of the government structure making it to chair by one of the ministers. Since then the number of the NGOs both national and international started to grow extensively reaching to 10,500 local NGOs and 94 international NGOs affiliated with SWC at present.

FUNCTIONING OF NGOS

Although the number of the NGOs, both national and international, increased extensively after the restoration of democracy in the country, they were not properly been regulated. Most of the international NGOs were left in confusion. They did not know what they can do and what they can not. Government policies could not come clearly in this context. Nor the laws and bylaws relating to NGOs and INGOs were made effective into their execution. Many things were left on adhoc basis. This adhocism further increased during the time of the collision government. Such a government proved itself worse in Nepal. Even the good people and the political parties were forced to turn out to be worse. As a result many of the INGOs were bound to go directly into implementation. They were also bound to find the door through which they can enter easily and get the support services required. Question of establishing the system and follow it up properly became secondary.

When INGOs were going directly into implementation, the issue of cost-effectiveness, sustainability and participation became futile. INGOs had to put more resources on salaries, benefits and overhead expenses which otherwise could have been reduced substantially had the programs been implemented through local NGOs. They also had to put extra resources for material and wages not knowing properly the local situations. Yet the outcome were moderate and, some times, they were ironic too, Likewise, sustainability of their activities in the field also limited to a larger extent into the slogan. When the INGOs pulled out after some years of their operation no alternative institutional mechanisms were redially available which could insure the continuity of the activities or keep on functioning the activities that were created. Nor it was possible to create new institutions in each and every situation within a limited period of time. Likewise the participation became misnomer. People (beneficiaries) were asked to contribute the labour and, often times, little cash. They were also asked to participate in the discussion during the time of project selection and sharing of benefits. But they were not involved in the crucial part of the activities i.e., management of the fund and the projects. This forced the people to consider the program as a gift and keep them on standing in distance with the expectation that everything will be provided by the project people. This created the sense of dependency and killed the spirit of the culture of local initiative.

Similarly local NGOs were left on their own. Once they were registered with the District Administration Office they could receive the funds from any source. They were not asked to formalize officially while receiving fund even from the foreign sources. Every one was virtually free to receive as well as give supports. Monitoring was almost nil and so was the case for evaluation on the part of the government institution. The local NGOs also were not particular to provide the progress report as well as audited statement of their accounts to the government institution. If they were to provide such reports they were giving directly to their funding agencies. The role of SWC, which was supposed to coordinate monitor and evaluate the NGOs' activities as well as promote and facilitate them on behalf of the government, was virtually inactive. Nor the relevant ministries of the government were positive to activate SWC effectively. Rather the contact ministry was even housed in the same building of SWC and the later was not spared to intervene in its operation. As a consequence NGOs were very much criticized by all concerns. They were criticized by the academicians, bureaucrats, general public and even by the NGOs themselves blaming one by other. Thus the entire situation was emerging as NGOs damizing in Nepal during the said period.

Realizing these things, since last two and a half years, some concrete steps on the part of SWC have been taken with the purpose of streamlining the entire sector and also to enhance its image. Among these steps the INGOs have been asked to work in partnership with local NGO without going themselves directly into implementation and provide whatever assistance they can do in terms of financial support, training facilities, technical assistance and information as well as knowledge sharing. They, however, have been allowed to enjoy freedom while selecting the partners and provide supports in the areas they like within the framework of the national priorities. It has also been started to categorize the INGOs into three groups depending upon their level of funding, working modalities and activities in consistence to the national policies. The type of visas and other facilities to be provided by the government have been proposed to be linked up with such categorization. Uniformity in agreement format, facility package, monitoring and evaluation as well in other requirements has started to bring into operation and no confusions have been allowed to remain without being clearly be defined.

As of the provision of the Social Welfare Act, local NGOs have strictly been asked to get the approval of SWC before receiving the fund from the foreign agencies. They have also been asked to maintain minimum requirements such as regular renewal of their registration, submission of progress report as well audited statement of their account every year and follow strictly their own constitution while presenting themselves as institution. If the local NGOs fail to fulfill these minimum requirements and get the approval while getting the foreign fund their registration will not be renewed, which means such NGOs will have little chance to get the fund from any public sources. They could also be taken several other actions if they fail to fulfil the above requirements.

As a result of these steps the efficiency in terms of cost effectiveness, sustainability and participation has started to be seen. It has also started to be seen the positive result in the fields. NGOs also have started to be more disciplined, responsible and transparent. Besides this, the resources have started to be recorded with SWC which the NGOs have utilized. From the national prospective, these steps have helped gradually to bring the entire NGO sector into a system and make them to follow the institutional norms. It has also helped the NGOs grow as a third sector and complement the government as well as private sector in their activities. Also these have helped to identify the individual NGOs in terms of their efficiency as well responsibility to the government institutions to adopt them as their partners for the execution of their activities at the grass roots levels.

CHALLENGES AHEAD

It has been seen that the number of NGOs is growing rapidly and the experienced and professional people are also gradually getting involved in this sector in Nepal. It has also been seen that several steps have already been taken and some are under way to streamline the sector aiming to transform it as a responsible sector. Still there are many challenges with this sector which have to be addressed to promote it fully as a responsible, result oriented and people based sector. These challenges are associated with the NGOs themselves, government institutions and the doners

Challenges to the NGOs

There are many challenges associated with NGOs themselves. These challenges are largely related to the issues of transparency-particularly to the financial transparency, discipline, internal democracy and performances.

So far the financial transparency is concerned, there is an allegation that NGOs are very much reluctant to disclose their budget to the beneficiaries with whom they have been working. They are also equally reluctant to let other know their salary structure of their personnel. This aspect is still confidential with INGOs. Even the staff within the same organization do hardly know the salary and benefits of one staff by others. This applies with many of such organizations. The case with the expatriate staff working with many INGOs is further confidential. Even the finance division and/or the accountants do hardly know the salary and benefits of such expatriate staff. Normally these staffs are paid directly at their country of origin and/or head office. This practice of paying the salary of expatriate staff in the country of origin has complicated the process of tracing down currently the real income of such staff and assess for income taxes for the governments of the concerned countries.

Concerning to the discipline and internal democracy, a large number of the NGOs are hardly appreciative to maintain the minimum requirements and follow the established norms. They are very prone to find out the easiest way to enter in and grab the opportunity even if that is contrary to the set principle. Likewise there are many local NGOs who have hardly made their membership opened and held election as defined in their own constitution. Often times, it has also been made the allegations that some of the NGOs are under the control of the family members, some have been created by the people in positions and still there are some NGOs created by INGOs and donor community to funnel out their supports.

There are also NGOs who produces plenty of paper works, make long speeches and publicize through seminars, workshops and several other media's. But their performances at the grass roots level effecting actually to the people are very limited. Yet they making their voices very strong. So the question is how to address these type of challenges. Should not the NGOs themselves be careful on this and address the issue of transparencies, discipline, internal democracy and result-based performances?

Challenges to the Government

Although the government in Nepal has NGO positive policy at present and it has recognized NGOs as its development partners but it has yet to facilitate to bring all NGOs and INGOs within one umbrella, cut-down the unnecessary steps for administrative efficiency and bring uniformity in support services. At present the NGOs, exclusively the INGOs, have been delt from different ministries as against the provision of the Social Welfare Act 1992 and the policies of the current five year plan of His Majesty's Government. This has made the monitoring of such INGOs' activities problematic and bring them into the uniform system of support services. At present these are differences in facilities provided by the government to the INGOs having agreement with different government institutions.

Similarly the administrative process within the government institutions are very lengthy and cumbersome. It has to travel several institutions each having too many steps to get the decision done in the matters of work permit, visa and agreement etc. This has, in fact, nothing to do but to waste time, energy and, often money too and create unnecessary burden to all parties concerned.

The question, therefore, rises how these problems could be addressed and bring all the NGOs within one umbrella, cut down the unnecessary administrative steps and bring uniformity in support services. Unless the government does this, it is hard to convince to the people that the government in practice is really committed towards its NGO positive policy and accepts the NGOs as one of its development partners.

Challenges to the Donors

NGOs in Nepal are mostly dependant to the donors for their funding. The donors also gradually are becoming positive to go through NGOs and civil societies for the channelization of their supports. However a large proportion of such supports have been lost in between the primary donors and target groups, since there are many organizations lined up on the way to primary donors and the target groups. The donors, therefore, have to find out the proper ways how this gap could be narrowed down between them and the target groups and bring more resources to the grass roots. If it is failed to do so it will subdue the very purpose of the donors assistance and also allow a ground to the people of both sides i.g. the tax payers/contributors in the donor countries as well as the beneficiaries in the recipient countries to raise a voice as against of this situation. Creating an environment through which a larger proportion of the supports could be brought down directly to the people at the grass roots level therefore, is a challenge to the primary donors.

Similarly the intermediary donors, especially the INGOs, are often times trying to create their own NGOs in Nepal and implement the activities through them when they were asked to go through local NGOs on partnership basis to avoid the problems of sustainability, participation and cost-effectiveness. This has created an unnatural situation and a conflict has emerged between the NGOs created and the NGOs spontaneously emerged. Likewise, the people working with the intermediary donor agencies as employees are also operating NGOs and are, often times, becoming donors as well as recipients themselves. This has given a ground to doubt to the people on such INGOs even if they do not have any bad intention with them. Therefore how to encounter these type of situations and create a fair environment removing unnecessary doubts and establishing mutual trust is another challenge to such intermediary donors.

SUMMARY AND CONCLUSIONS

We saw from this discussion that all civil societies are not NGOs. They need to possess certain characteristics to be called themselves NGOs. These characteristics are that they should be development oriented, non-political non-profit making and democratic in characters.

Viewing from these prospectives, the growth of NGOs started quite late in Nepal. Still the speed has increased rapidly from 1979 and by now the number of local NGOs has reached to 10,500 and INGOs to 94 affiliated with Social Welfare Council, a government organization dealing with NGOs in Nepal.

Despite this sudden growth in number, NGOs are doing good jobs in many respects. They have become effective especially in ares of awareness raising, organizing people into various functional groups, sharing of information and linking such groups with various service agencies. These activities also are noticeable in the fields of activating the people in agriculture, livestock rearing, community forestry, sanitation, drinking water supply, child care, health education, functional literacy and saving and credit cooperatives etc. Some of the NGOs are also doing commendable jobs in the delivery of health services, particularly the eye care as well as general health services. Still the NGOs have been heavily criticized due to the reasons of not being themselves regulated and communicated there activities properly.

Realizing these things, SWC at present is trying to regulate the NGOs and bring them into the system. It is also trying to make them more disciplined, responsible and democratic. But they have yet to do many things. They have to be fully transparent and result based. They have also to be accommodative to keep their membership open and act strictly according to their own constitution. Likewise the INGOs also are needed to be more cost effective, participatory and sustainable for their activities. For this there is no other option than to work on in partnership basis with high sincerity and honesty.

On the part of the government it should try to bring all NGO within one umbrella and remove the administrative constrains caused by the on-going lengthy process. It should also try to bring uniformity in the matters of support services and bring a clear cut policies while providing financial supports as well tax concessions. Till these days the government is missing to pay the attention and create an environment which can encourage the business houses and the general public for the support of the NGOs on financial basis.

Similarly, the primary donors also should be careful in the matters of creating their own NGOs in an artificial way and try to find out the alternative ways to cut down too many layers between the primary donors and real beneficiaries. Failing to do this the intermediary agencies will keep on benefiting in the name of the poors and the disadvantaged from the supports of the donors as it is happening at present.

Hence all the stockholders - the donors, government and the NGOs themselves, have to change their behaviors and adopt corrective measures if the NGOs have to be present as an effective, responsible and people-based sector. Missing to do this, there is a possibility that instead of supporting to the NGOs many of the behaviors that are in practice at present may damage the image of this sector and that will make difficulty for the NGOs to justify their presence itself.

6. UNDERSTANDING VOLUNTARY ACTION IN NEPAL

Diwakar Chand

HISTORICAL PERSPECTIVE

Observation of the evolutionary pattern of social services reveals that voluntary action occupied a very significant role in the overall development of social services in Nepal. There were traditional establishments which made an effort to consolidate and mobilise voluntary actions specially the *Guthis*, the systems of *Parma* and *Dhiku'* etc. *Guthi* is considered to be one of the most effective forms of delivering social services through an organised and scientific manner whereby the voluntary actions are optimally utilised. Although a *Guthi* has a limited outreach and are found (in most of the instances) grouping in and around several family households belonging to a particular ethnic groups this model over a period of time has proven its impact and efficiency. The *Guthis* are solely operated by *Guthiyars* who willingly volunteers to contribute his/her voluntary action to the members of the *Guthiyars* and to the *Guthi* itself whenever it is called for. However the outreach of the Guthis are found mostly concentrated towards the maintenance ,preservation and development of shrines and temples that has been built through the voluntary actions of the *Guthiyars*, extend support to the *Guthiyars* during the time of their need ranging from the birth of a child till performing the final funeral rites.

Similarly the practice of *Parma* which is still prevalent in the hilly and mountainous districts of Nepal stresses the importance of voluntary action . The voluntary action which is very similar to the concept of labour par theory stresses the exchange of voluntary action for farming purposes only. All the households in the Villages (where these practices are prevalent) are expected to render voluntary action to till the farm of the member of the households of the village on a rotational basis. This practice is still prevalent in several hilly and mountainous district of the country even till now.

The other forms of voluntary action that needs to be described here is the concept of *Dhikur* which is very popular amongst the Thakali community of Northern mountainous regions of Nepal. The *Dhikur* is very similar to the concept of micro credit where by the Members of the *Dhikur* are voluntarily extended credit to undertake prospective enterprises. This practice is , also confined and limited only within this community and to the members only[1].

---

[1] 'Development Through Non-Governmental Organisation', Diwakar Chand, p.15.

65

Although voluntary action has been occupying an integral part in the social development of the country since time immemorial, institutionalisation of voluntary action seemed to have taken roots only during the later part of the 19th century. As early as in 1895 Madhav Raj Joshi under the influence of Swami Dayananda sowed the seed of 'Arya Samaj' in Nepal which can be safely considered as one of the first process of institutionalising voluntary action to socially and spiritually liberate the community by generating awareness against the cruelty being imposed in the name of religion. The reformist movement steered by Mr. Joshi had a far reaching consequences in the society which is still being felt even till today in Nepal.

Similarly , the 'Charka Movement ' initiated by Mahatma Gandhi in India was replicated by Tulsi Meher in Nepal,who is lauded to be one of the first individual to initiate 'Charka Prcaharak Sanshthan' whose ulterior objective was to generate awareness and consolidate voluntary action from the community who at the time was being subjected to social and political subjugation by the then autocratic Rana rulers. Consolidation of voluntary action as the consequence of the awareness being generated by these individuals led to the establishment of 'Paropakar Samshthan' in 1947 which is effectively functional even till today.

CONTEMPORARY STATUS

While deliberating on the issues of institutionalisation of voluntary action in the context of Nepal effort here is made to analyse and evaluate only those sectors and institutions whose formative structure is largely voluntary in nature specially the Non-Governmental Organisation (NGOs) ,Community Based Organisations (CBOs) and Self Help Groups.

NGO is defined as an independent(entirely and/or largely), free from Government (World Bank's views), non-profiteering, autonomous, legally established, voluntary social organisation. Vertical growth of NGOs is being witnessed after the Peoples Movement of 1991. It is estimated that from a mere size of 219[2] in 1991 the size now has grown to 8325[3]. However the size is much bigger when we take into account those NGOs registered with CDOs and those not retaining affiliation with the Social Welfare Council(SWC) is said to be roughly around 15.000.[4]

It is mandatory for those registered under the Societies Registration Act of 1977 to have a minimum membership of seven individuals to retain legitimacy to register NGO. Most of the NGOs after having registered usually have a tendency of raising the size of members largely with a view of physically and materially

---

[2] Social Services National Coordination Council, 1990.

[3] Social Welfare Council, March 1998.

[4] This has been stated in the presentation by Dr. Tika Pokharel, member-secretary of the Social Welfare Council in a forum of 'NGO-Governmental Organisation in Development' organised by Central Department of Public Administration, March 19th, 1999.

strengthening the institution. Most of these NGOs have a provision for open membership whereby they encourage enhancing and enlarging the size of the members. It should be realised here that in most of the cases the major internal source of resource generations by these NGOs are accomplished through the membership fees which although may be nominal but poses a significant part of the contribution and possess sentimental value.

Since NGOs in Nepal is largely a voluntary social organisation, voluntary action occupies a very significant position towards the development pattern of these organisation. It is estimated that out of the total size of 8000 plus NGOs 16 of them retain a national status. National status based NGOs are usually defined as those which has operational entities and/or some forms of networking in almost all the 4 Development Regions of the country. Conservative estimate reveals that the total voluntary strength of these 16 NGOs alone is around 6,74,078(please see ANNEX-1).It would therefore be safe to predict that the voluntary strength associated with the NGOs in Nepal should be somewhere around 1 million. Services to be delivered and messages to be advocated by these retinue of volunteers if properly administered will definitely have a far reaching 'effect in the national development context of the country.

FORMATIVE STRUCTURE OF VOLUNTARY ACTION IN NEPAL

It should be properly analysed as to what would be the built-in strength of these NGOs and where and how their voluntary action could be creatively and productively mobilised to seek optimum results.

When we talk of NGOs we are basically talking of the greater stalk of NGOs who are registered with the Chief District Officers under the Societies Registration Act and we usually tend to undermine those professional enterprises registered as NGOs under the Company Act 2053(1995) according to which "With an objective to earn profit any person individually and/or collectively are entitled to open a Company with a single and/or several objective"[5] The Company Registration act enables any individual to open a Company either under single proprietorship and/or private limited company with one and/or more directors. Similarly to undertake a public limited Company it requires at least seven directors.

Therefore when we look at the formative structure of NGOs specially while delving upon voluntary action it would do more justice just to take into account those registered with the CDOs. These NGOs are registered 'as voluntary organisation motivated to deliver social services mostly to the downtrodden, needy and socially exploited segment of the community without any profiteering objective'. The basic premises under which most of these NGOs are built are mostly on a strong 'welfare-base' with an ulterior objective of

---

[5] See Article 2,Clause 3 of Company Act 2055.

delivering altruistic ,philanthropic and charity based services. Deliverance of such services mostly required retinue of dedicated volunteers and supportive logistic resources. Combination of these two ingredients was deemed to be sufficient to initiate NGO operation adequately. These NGOs even till date are overwhelmingly built upon the 'welfare base' and merely possess a large retinue of voluntary action force. Their voluntary action has definitely proven to be effective in the sectors of disabilities, special education, poverty alleviation, health and environment awareness generation, family planning etc.

A study by the World Bank[6] makes an observation that "the sociological concept of " voluntary organisations applies to NGOs in developing countries, but sometimes this concept is defined by sociologists in a narrow manner, so as to include "not-for-profit" characteristic. But the realm of NGO has expanded tremendously.

DEMAND FOR CHANGING ROLE OF VOLUNTARY ACTION

NGOs are being demanded to deliver not only social services but they are being increasingly demanded to cater 'developmental goods' as well. The 9th five-year plan explicitly refers to the NGOs as development agent "Enable to promote NGOs as partners of development and to make their programme more effective, coordinated effort is anticipated to be taken"[7].

It even goes further whereby it elucidates that "In the overall context of development the role of NGOs shall be assessed where by their participation in sectors like poverty alleviation,economic and social development shall also be incorporated in the policy document" The 9th plan specifically stresses that "NGOs shall be given priority in those sectors where they have gained specialisation even if such projects are being operated by the government and/or local entities".

The challenges that NGOs are to face now are more competitive and demanding than in the past. It needs to reshape itself from the conservative definition of 'values driven voluntary organisations 'to a 'developmental driven NGOs'. This altogether requires more than a retinue of volunteers. It demands for intervention, involvement and participation of 'professionals' skilled manpower and trained volunteers . The sectors where NGOs are basically involved are largely as follows:

1. Child Welfare
2. Health sector
3. Handicapped and disability
4. Community Development

---

[6] 'Nongovernmental Organisations and Local   Development', Michael M.Cernea, The World Bank,Washington DC, 1988, p.14.
[7] '9th Plan- Base Paper', National Planning Commission, 1998, p.33-34.

5. Women development
6. Youth Activities
7. Morel development
8. Environment protection
9. Education
10. Aids and drugs

STRATEGIES FOR MORE PRODUCTIVE MOBILISATION OF VOLUNTARY ACTION

All of these sectors demand extensive voluntary action, but that all by itself is not enough. More effective delivery of even these services demands for greater skills and more professional intervention . This therefore reveals a need for a two pronged strategies:

- It would require existing NGOs to extensively reorient, upgrade and enhance its capacity by rendering skilled based training programme and thereby adopt them more towards the delivery of 'development goods and/or

- Create new facilities and develop altogether new genes of development oriented NGOs.

Both of these strategies have pluses and minuses. With regard to the first strategy it is less time consuming largely because the structure and premises are already there where as in the second scenario altogether a new premises needs to be set up consumes more time.

NGO if it ever anticipates to enhance its efficacy and make optimum utilisation of the asset it possess in forms of voluntary action it needs to act with more seriousness and it has to take the decision now. No body is challenging the NGOs for not being able to reach out to the poor and the needy, nor are they being questioned for not delivering the services at the grassroots level. But what is being questioned is not being able to deliver 'effectively' and not being able to reach out the grass root level in a qualitative manner. This has led the entire credibility of NGOs being challenged at several quarters. So what needs to be done is to chalk out effective and pragmatic strategies to steer the voluntary action of the NGOs more productively.

PROPOSED MEASURES

1. Development of a Multideciplinary Resource Centre(MRC): The basic thrust and function of MRC shall be to largely to act as an institution to provide information, training and even counselling to the NGOs in sectors where NGOs involvement and intervention are pertinent. The formation of MRC could either be altogether a new entity established to build the capacity of the NGOs ranging from professional to technical skills and/or make an effort to

'pool-in' professionals and experts from in and around the like minded NGOs to perform this function.

2. There are quite a number of International Voluntary Organisations(IVO)s working in Nepal their expertise also could be shared to a certain extent.

3. Establishment of Trade Schools and Training centres with specific focus to train the volunteers associated with NGOs specially in the field of health, education, drinking water, sanitation, environment, income generation etc.

4. Set up a Volunteer Bank which will be entirely based upon time sharing concept.

5. Initiate undertaking formal NGO courses with a provision to render certificates and/or even degrees on NGOs.

6. Create new and prospective opportunities and venues for effectively and productively mobilising Voluntary action.

When we talk of volunteers specially in the social sector the connotation that is being used is slightly different from the definition being used in other parts of the world. A 'Volunteer' and 'voluntarism' in Nepali term would specially refer to rendering of services voluntarily without anticipating any benefits and or returns. There is absolutely no benefits and/or material incentive involved in the celibate definition of Voluntarism and voluntary action in Nepalese context. The existing practices of most of the IVOs are such that there is a built-in provision to provide allowances(off course subsidised),visa fees are gratis, vehicles (supportive personal commuters), lodging facilities and logistic support are usually provided. Under such circumstances it would appear to be a privilege for social workers to be a volunteer if this definition was to be applied.

If we are to learn to speak the language of the third generation volunteers we may have to gradually introduce the western notion of allocating subsidised budget for the services being provided by the volunteers. In this context it should be cautioned that" No responsible donor should undertake to "assist" or "use" NGOs to help in development unless it is prepared to invest in understanding their nature and distinctive roles. Financial incentives, wrongly applied, can destroy the voluntarism of all but the most strongly self-aware of voluntary organisations"[8].

UNDERSTANDING VOLUNTARY ACTION: NGOS PERSPECTIVE

NGOs are the single largest sector which tends to use and mobilise the voluntary action to the optimum which is closely followed by CBOs.The nature and pattern of voluntary actions being used and implied by these institutions differs from NGOs to CBOs and even from NGOs to NGOs. Since NGOs are largely voluntary organisations they are optimally by volunteers. Very few local NGOs

---

[8] 'Understanding Voluntary Organisations-Guidelines for Donors', L. David Brown & David C.Korten,World Bank,1989

although may have the provision but they don't seem to have the capacity to have well paid full time professional staffs. Since most of the volunteers associated with these NGOs work with no budget and/or have no provision for budget and/or even if they have provision they don't have the supportive resources to pay them, it has become rather very difficult for NGOs to retain 'professionals' within the institution.

Some of the NGOs specially those who are fairly large do have professional volunteers but they have not been able to tap them adequately. Due to these reasons Voluntary action does seem to have broadening effect mostly in the social service sector where as its effect in the development sector still is not prominent.

When we speak of fairly large NGOs, most of them are donor driven. In spite of their mixed manning pattern the major proportion of their budget for the paid professional staffs and most of the administrative expenses are born through external assistance. It should be cautioned here that if the donors ceases to participate there is every possibility for such NGOs to entirely collapse this applies to most of the donor driven NGOs in Nepal with very few exception. The irony is that the voluntary action all by itself cannot sustain and safeguard the very existence of these NGOs. We need to develop models which are not donor prone and which can be steered and sustained solely through the effort of voluntary action. This would demand for effective and dedicated strategies in the domestic frontier which calls for:

1. First of all the NGOs should mobilise voluntary action to raise and harness internal resources to the optimum and reduce the level of dependency upon external resources. This cannot be accomplished overnight. It is a time consuming process which calls for a lot of patience and dedication.
2. There has to be more amiable environment and understanding   between the government and the NGOs. The Government should specifically demarcate the grey area for NGOs involvement and participation.
3. National plan of action for the NGOs should be chalked out in the National policies and in the national document of the Government.
4. Once the role of NGOs in the national development context has been defined, supportive budget should also be allocated which should be entirely based upon the credibility, strength and built-in voluntary strength and action of the NGOs.
5. If voluntary action is to be diverted towards development activities the NGOs should also make all the effort to be more transparent and accountable.
6. More enduring and stable solidarity should be built amongst NGOs Collective consensus regarding pertinent NGO issues should be reached and they should be able to develop a forum to resound the issues and safeguard

the rights of the NGOs. This would call for mobilisation of collective voluntary action on behalf of the NGOs.

7. Productive mobilisation of Voluntary action would also call for developing a pragmatic Inventory of NGOs inclusive of the size and pattern of their voluntary strength.

8. Effort should be made and mechanism should be built towards more frequent co-sharing of volunteers amongst NGOs.

CBOS PERSPECTIVE

There are thousands of volunteers associated with CBOs as well. It is increasingly being felt by many social delivery agency's that it is more convenient to work with CBOs in the rural areas rather than undertake the execution on their own shoulders. This has led to mushrooming growth of CBOs in Nepal The voluntary action associated with these sectors have proven to be very effective and active. The association of voluntary actions are mostly in forms of users group and/or consumer forums. Using voluntary action in these sectors have proven that the question of sustainability is more pragmatically addressed than in the NGO mechanism. The CBOs seem to have more stronger sense of belongings than the NGOs and they seem to be more intricately attached and fabricated with the forums which gives them more jurisdiction and also more sense of responsibility which seem to be strongly lacking in NGOs mechanism.

The status of CBOs are both formal and non-formal. Most of the CBOs are found maintaining registrations with different Governmental Line Agency's (GLA) and therefore such CBOs retain formal status. Where as there are CBOs who have been functioning as users group and/or consumers groups but have as yet not retained any affiliation with any GLAs as such. A conservative estimate conjectures the total strength of CBOs are somewhere around 25,000[9].

The formative structure of CBOs reveal that amongst those who are most active are the Irrigation Canal Consumers Committee (ICCC) closely followed by Community Forest Consumers Committee (CFCC).With regard to ICCC they have been established for quite sometime and therefore retains the largest number memberships. CFCC is gaining a great deal of popularity after the government started initiating the transfer and conversion of state owned forest to community ownership. The community ownership forest are being administered, managed and monitored by the community who have been delegated with the authority. They have taken the entire responsibility of nurturing and conserving the delegated forest by manning their volunteers and they have even been authorised to impose fines and punish the culprits who are found guilty of trying to harm and/or destroy the forest in any ways. They set up a public court in the concerned village and settle the dispute there and then. They have been given the

---

[9] Nepal Consumers Federation, March 1999.

rights and discretion to even share the forest-by products and retain the portion of the earnings for their upkeep. There are even instances specially with regard to those forest lots which are declared as 'dillipated' where the consumer committee members are given the opportunity to preserve that portion of the vegetation that can be saved and the rest of the area can be cultivated and/or used for farming.

The advantage of CBOs as against NGOs are that the formative structure of CBOs are such that they are the larger and/or ultimate beneficiary of the project they are involved in. The intrinsic strength of such 'self-help' groups and their project is that if anything goes wrong with the project they are going to be the ultimate looser. They therefore make it a point to put in their entire energy and input to make the project successful. They seem to have proven the strength of voluntary action. A country which was being incriminated with the charges of amassing almost one hectare of forest per annum is being managed and protected through the voluntary actions of the CFCCs. I strongly feel that the most successful case study that one can confidently project with regard to the productive mobilisation of voluntary action is that of CFCCs.

It is therefore not disputable that if we make an effort to properly understand the voluntary action and if we endeavour to make best use of them the country at large could reap the direct benefit accruing from it. If the voluntary action is not properly mobilised and if it remains unrecognised and unnoticed, it would not just be a great loss to the nation but it would also lead to the peril of sowing unforeseen dangers that may possibly arise from a battalion of ideal and unemployed mass of voluntary action.

7. VOLUNTARY ACTIONS AND ETHNICITY IN NEPAL: CHALLENGES AND LIMITATIONS[1]

Krishna B. Bhattachan

Globally Nepal is in the "South" and we have both "North" and "South" within the country. My following views are, therefore, based on my experience living in the "South" of the "South"-life-world.

INDIGENOUS VOLUNTARY ACTIONS IN NEPAL: AN OVERVIEW

Voluntary actions in Nepal are as old as the indigenous ethnic groups themselves. It has been a way of their every-day-lives. Some of the outstanding indigenous voluntary organizations include *Dhikur* (rotating credit association) and *Dharma Panchayat* (local level political organization) among the Thakalis, *Guthi* (land based religious organization) of the Newars, *Rodi* (social organization) and *Ama Samuha* (mother's groups) of the Gurungs, *Bheja* (social, cultural, religious, political and economic organization) of the Magars, *Kipat* (communal land tenure system of the Limbus), *Khel* (socio-cultural organization) and the *Chattis Mauja* Irrigation system of the Tharus and *Parma* (labor exchange system) among various ethnic groups (for detail see Bhattachan 1996; 1997).

The main features of indigenous voluntary organizations are:

community based,
seasonal and temporary,
no official or legal recognition,
voluntary membership,
leadership based on seniority,
extensive use of local resources,
concern and priority to help disadvantaged individuals/families,

small group size,
less formal structure,
no formal rules and regulations,
decisions made through mutual consultation and agreement,
extensive use of indigenous knowledge, and
effective and sustainable.

If we evaluate these indigenous voluntary organizations by applying five attributes of success of induced voluntary organizations suggested by Aloyous P. Fernandez (1987), these indigenous organizations are successful because they too carry the attributes of success such as homogeneity, smallness, voluntaristic, participatory and non-political.

---

[1] This is a revised version of my paper presented in a dialogue seminar 'Voluntarism: Experiences and Reflections' organized in Kathmandu, Nepal by the Center for the Study of Developing Scoieties, New Delhi, and Coalition for Environment and Development, Finland in April 4-5, 1999.

All these indigenous voluntary actions indeed help to strengthen social economy and socio-cultural diversity very effectively and sustainably.

Before the territorial "unification" of Nepal by King Prtihvi Narayan Shah, who is regarded by some Nepalese as a "Gurkha imperialist," various nationalities had their own autonomous rules where voluntarism was the only rule of the game. Since 1768, King Prithvi Narayan Shah began his project of making Nepal an *Asali Hindustan* ("Real India" implying that *Hindustan* or India is "fake"), began to hit with a barrage of cultural Tomahawk missiles such as Hinduization, Sanskritization and *Bahunbad* (Brahaminism) targeted to various nationalities. Junga Bahadur Rana, the founder ruler of 104-year old autocratic Rana regime, promulgated the National Code of Nepal in 1854 by incorporating indigenous peoples within the caste hierarchy and making provisions of differential punishment based on who belongs where in the hierarchy. Fortunately, due to the lack of transportation and communication system, indigenous voluntary activities did not get extinct or badly damaged, though it declined gradually. Since 1950, indigenous voluntary activities has been resisting two powerful forces, one coming through the process of globalization and another coming through the intensification of the process of domination of one caste (Bahun-Chetri), one language (Nepali), one religion (Hindu) and one culture (Hindu) by the predatory Nepalese state. During the 30 years of autocratic Panchayat rule from 1960 to 1990, indigenous peoples were not even allowed to go for a picnic.

Although Nepal has been a multi-ethnic, multi-lingual and multi-religious country from time immemorial, the Bahun-Chetri rulers have never recognized this reality since the so-called "unification" (territorial unification) in 1768. During the last 230 plus years the predatory state has been imposing one-caste, one language, one religion, and one culture policy in the socio-culturally diverse society. Even the new "democratic" constitution of Nepal promulgated in 1990 declares Nepal as a Hindu Kingdom and discriminates between Nepali language and other 125 mother tongues and dialects. Though the Constitution of the Kingdon of Nepal, 1990 itself is very communal favoring Hindu religion and Nepali language, any voluntary activities done by the nationalities in social, cultural, religious and linguistic spheres has always been labeled as "communal", "anti-national", "divisive," "disintegrative" and "secessionist" by the ruling power elites.

Such a hopeless situation has changed somewhat since July 1997. The National Committee for Development of Nationalities (NCDN) was established by His Majesty's Government of Nepal under the Ministry of Local Development (MLD) in July 1997. The Committee has identified 61 nationalities in Nepal. This is the only committee within the government that has targeted to benefit the nationalities. The current Ninth Development Plan (1997-2002) made public in 1998 has given first ever long-term and five-year policies, plans and programs specifically for the indigenous and nationality groups in the country. Also, various national political parties, including the Nepali Congress, the Nepal Communist Party (UML), the Nepal Communist Party (ML), the Rastriya Prajatantra Party (Thapa), the Rastriya Prajatantra Party (Chand), the Nepal Sadvabana Party, the Nepal Majdoor Kisan Party, the Samyukta Jana Morcha (Sherchan), the Nepal Communist Party (Maoist) etc. have promised to do something for various nationalities in preserving, promoting and developing their language, culture, religion and economic conditions. Therefore, it is now no more a taboo to pursue nationalities-centered development policies, plans and programs by the governmental, non-governmental organizations and the donors. Even then, there are some bigot, fundamentalist Hindus, who do not hesitate to charge people with any such efforts as "anti-national" and "disintegrative."

So far we have witnessed four patterns concerning voluntary organizations and nationalities. These are:

1. Indigenous voluntary organizations of the nationalities;
2. Modern Nationality Organizations (such as the Nepal Federation of Nationalities (NEFEN) and its affiliated organizations;
3. NGOs run by either Bahun-Chetris or mixed groups with a domination of Bahun-Chetris and subordination of few individuals belonging to nationality groups and targeted to the development of various nationalities; and
4. NGOs run by the nationalities themselves.

(I)NGOs AND VOLUNTARY ORGANIZATIONS OF NATIONALITIES: IN THE PAST AND PRESENT

During the 30-year of autocratic partyless Panchayat political regime, that is, before the people's movement of 1990, voluntary organizations of various Nationalities were not allowed to work for any kinds of political or organized activities. However, some voluntary cultural organizations of some Nationalities such as the *Tharu Kalyankari Sabha* (Tharu Welfare Organization) of the Tharus, the *Nepal Tamang Ghedung* (Nepal Tamang Association) of the Tamanags, the *Thakali Sewa Samiti* (Thakali Welfare Committee) of the Thakalis and *Cwasa Pasa* (Friend's Association) of the Newars have been active in cultural and linguistic spheres since the early fifties. Interestingly many voluntary cultural organizations of various Nationalities, including Rai, Limbu, Sunuwar, Yakkha Chhumma, Dhimal, Sherpa, Chhantyal, Rajbanshi, Chepang and Hyolmo sprouted in the eighties. After the people's movement of 1990 and reinstatement of multi-party political system, all these Nationalities formed the*Nepal Janajati Mahasangh* (Nepal Federation of Nationalities) [NEFEN] in 1990 with the objectives of coordinating these Nationalities to generate movements so as to regain their cultural, language and religious rights. NEFEN has so far demanded for ethnic autonomy, use of mother tongue in education at all levels and in the government owned electronic media, secularism, customary rights and transformation of the

Upper Hose into the House of Nationalities, and so on. NEFEN has pursued "movement approach" as opposed to "project approach."

Before the set up of the National Committee for Development of Nationalities (NCDN) in 1997, His Majesty's Government of Nepal (HMG-N) never recognized the existence of various nationalities in the country. As stated earlier, the predatory Nepali state has been pursuing a policy of one language (Nepali), one religion (Hindu), one culture (Hindu) and one dress for a long time. Such a policy has caused rapid destruction of various mother tongues (125 languages and dialects), religions and cultures.

Donors, including INGOs entered Nepal since the fifties. During the 30 years of autocratic partyless Panchayat rule, the rulers deterred donors and INGOs in pursuing development strategy geared to directly benefit various disadvantaged caste groups and nationalities. Some government officials maintain that they suggest donors and INGOs to help the poor and villagers living in remote areas but if the donors show their interest to implement programs for any specific caste or nationality, they strongly discourage them in doing so. Also, the donors believe that caste and nationality issue is the internal politics of Nepal and it is not ethical on their part to do something about it. Till now, unfortunately donors have, largely, abstained from pursuing caste and nationalities-centered development strategy.

The late King Mahendra had renamed the Chepangs as "Praja" and provided some fund for their upliftment. Since then HMG-N has allocated some budget every year for their development but research after research has revealed that the money is misused by the bureaucrats; so Chepangs have hardly benefited from it. Also, the Chepangs would like to identify themselves as Chepangs but not as "Praja."

Mr. Dilli Chaudhary, a young and energetic Tharu from Western Nepal, has been running a NGO called Backwards Society Education (BASE) since 1985 with international support to implement various programs for the upliftment of the Tharus in the Dang district in Western Nepal. According to Odegaard (1999:66) "Self-help through education is the main message of the BASE ideology" and by 1993, with DANIDA's support, "It has become the biggest local NGO in Nepal, working in 6 districts of West Nepal, with 100,000 members, 18,500 students and running 730 night classes in 325 villages in the districts of Dang, Banke, Bardiya, Kanchanpur, Kailali and Salyan." Mr. Chaudhary was awarded 1994 Reebok Human Rights Award in New York. Dilli's critic accuses BASE for its leader- or Dilli-centered approach. Odegaard (1999:82) has noted, "One problem faced by many NGOs is the danger of being taken over by and ruled by international NGOs (INGOs)" and "The pressure exerted on Dilli and BASE by politicians, foreign donors and locals, relatives and friends has led to a problem for Dilli regarding trust."

Four years ago, Plan International had helped the *Nepal Tamang Ghedung*, one of the active members of the National Federation of Nationalities (NEFEN), to implement some literacy programs in Tamang language and community child center in Makawanpur district. During those years, altogether 75 literacy classes and 24 child centers were established; 2 text books, 1 picture book, 1 guide book and 1 training manual were prepared. Last year the partnership stopped due to an unfortunate unprecedented problem. Initially the program did very well but later some greedy Tamangs came in the local level *Tamang Ghedung* who embezzled with the money that was supposed to be given for the Teachers. Also, writing or memo- and report culture of the INGO and oral culture of nationalities like *Tamang Ghedung* was also a problem for smooth communication between the two partners. However, the positive sides of the partnership include the transformation of oral tradition to written one, experience by the advocacy groups to run programs. Also, the local Tamangs liked the textbooks that were sensitive to their language, culture and tradition. The program indeed succeeded to attract a large number of the Tamangs in literacy classes. Unfortunately, weakness in financial management badly hampered the partnership. This is an unfortunate as well as an exceptional case.

Similarly, *Kirant Yakthung Chumlung* (Kirant Limbu Association) of the Limbus is supported by SIDA, a Canadian INGO, to run literacy classes in *Srinjanga* script and Limbu language. Also, Danish INGO MS-Nepal also helps the *Chumlung* to run some programs. Another INGO helps *Chumlung* to run rehabilitation programs for the drug addicts.

The SCF (USA) has been interested in helping the Dalits, nationalities and other disadvantaged groups and the CARE-Nepal, in its Strategy Paper has defined and identified disadvantaged groups (DAG) that includes the Dalits, nationalities, women and children. They have not been yet working with the organization of the nationalities.

During an informal conversation, a senior scholar associated with a reputed INGO working in Nepal told me that the INGOs are interested to work with voluntary organizations of indigenous ethnic groups but they have discovered that they are "too hot." Indeed they are "hot" because they are fully aware that if they cultivate association with (I)NGOs with a "project approach" they strongly believe that their "cause" of the resinstatement of their rights set back. Instead, if they strongly pursue a "movement approach" then it would definitely help to achieve their goal of egalitarian society.

(I)NGOS AND NATIONALITIES: PROSPECTS

So far INGOs and donors appears to have realized very seriously that they should pursue Dalit and nationalities-centered development strategy but as they are suggested by the government officials that such approach would be considered as violation in the internal political affairs of the country, they mostly have shied away from taking any initiative in this direction. Both donors and INGOs may take advantage of the NCDN and the Ninth Development Plan to move in this direction.

So far, NGO, that is induced NGO, has not yet infected nationalities. The current image of NGO in the country is very much tarnished, though there are handful of NGOs doing very good (Bhattachan 1998b; and Siwakoti "Chintan" 2056). At least, nationalities have not contributed for the current plight of NGOs. If most of the NGOs should continue such trend in future too, nationalities believe that it is better not to have any NGO than having rotten ones. Such a hopeless situation itself is an opening for improving the images of NGOs. As the nationalities are clean stated, if NGOs engage themselves working in partnership with various nationalities by engaging in advocacy in realizing "ethnic autonomy" or "right to self determination." It is an irony that most of the activists belonging to various nationalities are charged by the Bahun-Chetri rulers and "Bigots" or Hindu fundamentalists, including some journalists, that they are releasing "venom" in the peaceful society with the help of "foreigners" or "foreign money" to destabilize the Nepalese society. All Nationalities believe that such voice itself constitutes "venom" and the need of the time is "anti-venom" injection. Therefore, INGOs and donors may supplement or complement the NCDN and the Ninth Development Plan to infuse anti-venom in the Nepalese society to make it healthy. This means, INGOs and donors should work together with nationalities in advocacy for the establishment of egalitarian ("*samatamulak Samaj*") society.

Nationalities have in no way contributed in now already tarnished image of NGOs or induced voluntary activities in Nepal. So far, nationalities are "virgin" as they have not been penetrated by induced NGOs or voluntary organizations. Nationalities would welcome INGOs/donors if they are willing to support them in advocacy in two fronts: one, in realizing ethnic autonomy or right to self determination and two, in promoting literacy programs, basic and primary education and higher education in mother tongues. In such partnership, they do not want to see INGOs/donors/NGOs using the strategies of trick-all-down or trick-from-bottom-up or trick-from-inside-out-and-outside-in. Nationalities do not want support in other sectors because of their belief that NGOs cannot deliver development. Also, they demand that HMG-N to recognize and universalize indigenous voluntary organizations for the common good.

REFERENCES

Bhattachan, Krishna B.1996: "Induced and Indigenous Self-Help organizations in the context of Rural Development: A Case Study of the GTZ Supported Self-Help Promotion programs In Nepal," in *Social Economy and National Development*, Edited by Horst Mund and Madan Kumar Dahal, Kathmandu: Nepal Foundation for Advanced Studies (NEFAS), and Friedrick Ebert Stiftung (FES), Germany, 1996.

Bhattachan, Krishna B. 1997: "People/Community-Based Development Strategy in Nepal," pp.100-148, in *Developmental Practices in Nepal*, Edited by Krishna B. Bhattachan and Chaitannya Mishra, Central Department of Sociology and Anthropology, Tribhuvan University, Kathamdnu in cooperation with Friedrich Ebert Stiftung (FES), Nepal Office, Kathmandu, 1997.

Bhattachan, Krishna B.1998a:"Globalization and Its Impact on Nepalese Society and Culture," pp.80-102, in *Impact of Globalization in Nepal*, Edited by Madan K. Dahal, Kathmandu: Nepal Foundation for Advanced Studies (NEFAS), and Friedrick-Ebert-Stiftung (FES), Germany, 1998.

Bhattachan, Krishna B.1998b"*NGO: Yatharthata ra Bhram,*" ("NGO: Reality and Deception"), pp.12-25 , *Bikas*, Year 7 No.11, Saun 2055 (1998). (Text in Nepali).

Siwakoti "Chintan", Gopal 2056: "NGOmarfat Bhairaheko Rajnaitik Hastachhep" ("Political Interference Through NGO"), pp.11-15, *Red Star*, Baisakh-Jestha 2056.

Fernandez, Aloyous P.1987:"NGOs in South Asia: People's Participation in Partnership," *World Development*. Volume 15. Special Issue.

Odegaard, Sigrun Eide 1999: "BASE and the Role of NGOs in the Process of Local and Regional Change," pp. 63-83, in Harald O. Skar (ed.), *Nepal: Tharu and Tarai Neighbours*, Kathmandu: EMR.

8. POLICY PERSPECTIVE OF NGO OPERATIONS IN NEPAL

Tek Nath Dhakal

INTRODUCTION

Normally, the nation states carry out their plans and priorities to deliver goods and services to their people. The government involves various development organizations in the state affairs to influence the pattern of development and quality of legal & political aspects in the following five areas:

- development policies;
- content of development programs;
- administrative capacity enhancement;
- choice of organizational channels for carrying out development programs; and
- overall level of available funding and the level of resource mobilization. (Riker: 16-20).

However, socio-cultural background of the country, level of external assistance and the degree of external intervention in the national economy nature and extent of economic and political crises in the country are some other factors which affect the developmental process. These intrinsic and extrinsic variables call for rethinking the governmental role in carrying out the development efforts.

There are different schools of thoughts to explain the role of the NGOs. According to *public goods theory* or the 'performance failure theory', NGOs exist to satisfy the residual unsatisfied demand for public goods in society (Weisbrod, B.A., 1988). When the government could not fulfil the public goods for all the people or serve all the interests at least in the minimum level, or often, intended level, people should have to find out their alternative organizations in the form of people's organization or NGOs. This situation arises if the society is more diverse and heterogeneous. James argues that the more heterogeneous a society, the more conducive it becomes for creating larger number of NGOs (James 1991: 23). Brown and Korton argue that 'a widely recognized failure of large-scale government bureaucracy is their inflexibility and conservatism'. This political form of state failure creates a situation in which NGOs emerge as innovative responses to novel problems, because of their abilities for experimentation and flexibility. (Brown and Korten: 1991, 47)

Another influential and related theory is the *contract failure theory*. When people find it difficult to perceive the sense of contract, they have to find out reliable agents to fulfil their needs. Therefore 'non-profit organizations' could be more reliable agents in such situation as the commercial firms may take more advantage of the consumer's ignorance. Brown and Korton argue that organizations might come into existence to be as remedies in case of the 'market failures' situations because markets tend to be 'especially vulnerable to failure in developing countries', (Brown and Korten, 1991: 48).

Esman and Uphoff and also Uphoff and Cohen in their works argued that NGOs play the role of local intermediaries to fulfil the 'organizational gap'. According to this model, local intermediary mobilizes the people to participate in government-initiated programs. NGO could be a potentially effective medium, which could be utilized in delivering services to the rural areas of the developing countries. In this way, NGOs are taken as alternative institutional framework through which the rural poor and socially disadvantaged groups are served in a better way than the traditional bureaucratic mechanisms (Esman and Uphoff 1984; Uphoff and Cohen 1979; Korten 1981).

NGOs can play an effective role in alleviating rural poverty and helping communities adapt to modernization, building vibrant civil societies and shaping their inter-relationship with the society, state, and international civil society. They can also contribute to social movements by empowering people and contributing to alternative discourses of development and democratization. (Fisher: 1997, 440-441). This shows that NGOs could have diverse roles from grassroots development to building of international relation.

Nepal has been struggling with poverty despite decades of planned actions. She has completed eight periodic plans (four decades) and is currently implementing the Ninth Plan (1997-2002). The socio-economic transformation is naturally a *Herculean* task as the country has been facing with a maze of socio-economic-politico problems. Nepal's position in Human Development Index (HDI) is 154 out of the 175 states in the world and sixth in the SAARC region (UNDP: 1997, 146-148).

The government may be highly constrained with rigid and often outmoded rules and regulations, vested political interests, apathy and lack of initiatives on the part of government employees, rampant corruption and procedural red-tapism. This situation demands for appropriate alternative institutional measures for mobilizing local resources and unleashing the forces of development in a coordinated manner to speed up socio-economic enhancement. The failure of government in tackling with the multifarious problems such as providing basic needs, awareness creation, delivery of health facilities and providing a better livelihood led to the search of alternative institutional mechanism in the early 1970s. The expansion of NGOs community could be an asset to complement development initiative taken by the government.

However, problems that need to be addressed with care are many such as pervasive poverty, massive unemployment and underemployment, sluggish growth in the overall economy, the rate inflation far in excess of the growth in income of an overwhelming majority, increasing trade deficit (about 17 percent of GDP), increasing debt burden and continual large budget deficit, increasing foreign aid-dependence and low level of utilization of domestic resources for productive investment. (Guru-gharana: nd, 83).

It is natural that the people want concrete, visible and substantive results. But the poverty is the outcome of various factors such as mass illiteracy, poor health, insufficient employment opportunities & the economic deprivation, and inefficiency and rampant corruption including lack of political and administrative commitment. Many people in the country have been fighting for survival as 42 percent of the total populace (some others think at least 50-60% is under absolute poverty) live below the absolute poverty (NPC: 1997, 1). Therefore, NGOs are taken as development partners for implementing the activities related to community and rural development, urban slums, empowerment of women, improvement of environment, delivery of public health, irrigation providing health education on AIDS and drug abuse, youth activities and development of moral values (NPC: 1992-97:569-572).

The role of NGOs in accelerating the pace of development and strengthening democracy is crucial in developing countries like in Nepal. In the changed political context, NGOs are expected to function as a catalyst, as mobilizers, facilitators, analysts and advocates of the people (Tuladhar 1991). As people get more opportunities in democracy for the attainment of self-governance, self-reliance and sustainable development, their organized efforts could play crucial role for furthering democracy also. Such roles become crucial because of their interdependence of local organizations and institutions, their functional specialization, their accountability to the people, etc. This could demand people's own initiatives to solve their problems. In this way people could create their organizations which call POs/NGOs, etc.

NGOs as new institutional mechanism have been considered as agent of resources transfer and implementation of aid programs in the development arena, which could either complement or supplement the governmental efforts. Apart from the public and private sector, the non-profit sector, i.e., NGO interventions are necessary in transforming the socio-economic condition of the people. As a result, this sector has explosively proliferated with increased involvement in various areas of public life, both local and national interests. However, there is an ongoing debate regarding NGO's role and impact. Some of the positive aspects advocated in favour of NGOs are related with their efficiency, cost effectiveness, flexibility and familiarity with grassroots problems, innovativeness, transparency in working procedure and more sincere dedication not guided by profit. Likewise, their approach to mobilizing people's participation and willingness to work with small groups are also held as positive attributes. At the other end of the spectrum, some of the negative attributes that often go with NGOs are institutional weakness, low level of resourcefulness, equipped, deficiency in infrastructure, lack of self-reliance and short-term considerations. They are also deficient in trained and professional manpower.

Recent issues and concerns of the people and the government both in the donor countries or institutions and recipient countries are related to the roles, institutionalization, voluntarism, transparency, cost effectiveness, and accountability of the NGOs. Due to the favourable policies adopted during the last three decades and particularly after 1990s NGOs in Nepal have excessively proliferated. But what about the consequences of that rapid growth and how the policy directives impact the NGO functions towards the socio-economic transformation are the basic issues today.

INSTITUTIONALIZATION OF NGO IN NEPAL

Institutionalization process of the social institutions has begun in Nepal in the late 1950s. As an endeavour, enactment of *Societies Registration Act, 1959* was the first independent initiative taken by the government to institutionalize this sector. This Act spelt out the domain, *modus operandi* and functioning procedures of the social organizations to some extent. Some other Acts that guided and supported the functions or registration of the NGOs were *Society Registration Act 1959; National Directives Act 1962; Muluki Ain* (Civil Law) 1962; and *Company Act & Regulations* 1965.

A change in the strategy of the OECD countries in the transfer of capital to the developing countries through NGO channels encouraged the creation of more and more NGOs in the developing countries like Nepal. This was coupled with the strategy changes of the World Bank and similar other international financial institutions. In this context, the government in association with the national level social workers held seminars in Rampur, Chitwan in 1971, Mujhelia, Janakpur in 1974 and again in Mujhelia, Janakpur in 1976 (Chand: 1998, 49-50). These seminars did a lot of homework to highlight the role of social organizations and classifying them in accordance with their discipline and sectoral affiliation. Until 1970s NGOs were required to maintain relations with concerned Line Ministries according to their functional discipline and sectoral affiliation as there was no uniformity in rules and regulations regarding the NGO operation in Nepal. A one-window policy for the operation of social organizations was subsequently felt for more enhanced and effective functioning of the NGOs. These seminars diagnosed such problems and suggested for a separate Act to govern the social organizations along with the creation of a central level organization for coordinating and facilitating the social organizations scattered in the country (Chand: 1991, 33-34).

Accordingly, in 1977, the government brought *Sangh Sangstha Ain 2034* (Organization and Association Act 1977) for the institutionalization of the social service institutions in Nepal. In the same year, the *Social Service National Coordination Council Act* also called *Samajik Sewa Ain* was enacted and Social

Service National Coordination Council (SSNCC) was established as a governmental bureau. The *Sangh Sangstha Ain 2034* covered all voluntary institutions while the *Samajik Sewa Ain* (Social Service Act) covered social welfare organizations authorized by SSNCC.

There were six coordination committees under the SSNCC. They were the Community Service Coordination Committee, the Youth Activity Coordination Committee, the Health Service Coordination Committee, the Child Welfare Coordination Committee, the Women Service Coordination Committee, and the Hindu Religion Service Coordination Committee. On the basis of activities the NGOs were categorized under any one of the Coordination Committees. The role of the SSNCC was to work as an umbrella organization for all the NGOs working in the country. This organization was supposed to work for the promotion, facilitation, co-ordination, monitoring and evaluation of the activities of the non-governmental organizations in Nepal. However, the social workers felt more suffocated and controlled by this centrally guided provision. That is why NGOs could not expand rapidly during the period of 1970s and 1980s.

Before 1990, various factors led to the expansion of NGOs. The normal practice was the requirement for NGOs to get registered with the *CDO office[1]* in order to get affiliated with the SSNCC. Many social organizations could not get registered until the local authority was fully assured of their loyalties to the existing political system. It was simply because the government which was always suspicious about the NGOs on political grounds, multiparty political activities by these NGOs being the most dreaded aspect. Therefore, NGOs were registered by CDO office after through investigation. During that period, mostly the Kathmandu-based elites could create NGOs. So, some 70% NGOs were working in Kathmandu while the rest 30% worked in the district headquarters. (Sob, 1991). Many NGOs were something like what Korten (1991) calls GONGOs. In order to avoid excessive government control, some NGOs circumvented these Acts by registering non-profit research institutions under the 1964 Company Act (Lama et.al. 1991:3).

Similarly other negative factor that contributed to the suppression of NGOs was a mandatory provision to get prior approval of the SSNCC for their registration. It was not practical to take prior approval from the Kathmandu based SSNCC for a person (s) of the district. Therefore the NGO workers at the grassroots and NGO sector specialists indicate that there was a deliberate attempt to restrict the growth of NGOs as the registration required time consuming screening procedures. Further NGOs were also not allowed to focus on development issues, which could sensitize the people to challenge their status quo in the social and political power structure. (CECI: 1992, 8).

---

[1] Chief District Officer (CDO) is the administrative head of each District Administration Office. Normally, NGOs should be registered in the CDO Office and could be affiliated with SWC Office.

Despite these anomalies regarding NGO operation creation of *Ministry of Labour and Social Welfare (MLSW)* in 1981 could be taken as an important step towards institutionalisation of social service sector in the kingdom. This institution has to work as a central level organisation for planning, policy formulation and implementation of social welfare and non-governmental functions. SSNCC was brought under this ministry. SSNCC needed to work in co-ordination with the Foreign Ministry for formal visa and the Home Ministry for non-tourist visa. Likewise, it works in co-ordination with the Finance Ministry for duty-free status and tax exemption. The Council also worked with he NPC for the co-ordination of NGO activities with national activities. Apart from them, there are other line ministries with whom the SWC worked together in concerned areas. They are Local Development Ministry, Ministry of Health, and Ministry of Population and Environment. According to the SWC Act the minister who looks after the MLSW (at present it has changed into Ministry of Women and Social Welfare since 1996) become the chairman of the council.

It is only after the restoration of democracy in 1990 that a congenial atmosphere for proliferation of NGOs has been created in Nepal. As an endeavor *Social Welfare Act 1992* was enacted and Social Welfare Council (SWC) replaced the existing SSNCC. Other Acts have also been enacted which are also related directly or indirectly with the social welfare works. Some of these Acts are *Village Development Committee Act 1992; Municipality Act 1992; District Development Committee Act 1992; Children's Act 1992; Cooperative Act 1993; Natural Disaster Relief Act 1993; and Handicapped Protection & Welfare Act 1993.*

After enactment of these Acts a new movement came in the NGO dynamism in Nepal. Some of the noticeable changes can be found as follows:

- Interested people could register any type of NGO in the CDO office after completing certain prescribed formalities, i.e., does not require any recommendation or prior approval from any other institute(s).
- Due to the enactment local bodies Act (such as District Development Committee Act the Municipality Act and Village Development Committee Act etc.), there was sufficient 'political space' for the NGO to stretch their activities and allowed to focus on development issues, which could sensitize the people to challenge their status in the social and political power structure..
- The channeling process of foreign resources through NGOs have been simplified, and make more convenient to transfer donor/INGO resources to the local partner and when tripartite agreement between donor, recipient NGO and the SWC would be taken place.
- Affiliation process was also made easier and mandatory to complete the process within a three months' period.
- The scope of mobilizing the local manpower and resource together with foreign resource has been felt easier.

POLICY IN THE EIGHTH PLAN (1992-97) AND NINTH PLAN (1997-2002)

Planned economic development effort started in Nepal since 1956. The objectives of the First Plan (1956-61) were to raise production, employment, standards of living and general wellbeing throughout the country. By the time the goals set for Sixth (1980-85) and the Seventh (1985-90) plans were fulfilling the basic needs of the people. The objectives of the Eighth Plan (1992-97) were "alleviation of poverty, sustainable economic growth and reduction of regional imbalance". The current Ninth Plan (1997-2002) has set a single objective of 'poverty alleviation'. The concept of long-term development has also been introduced in 1997. The long-term development objective is to create a society that is cultured, modern, development-oriented and endowed with skills through alleviating the prevailing wide spread poverty in the country (NPC: 1998, 59). However, the planned efforts could not make much impact on the socio-economic lives as the majority of the people are still fighting with a host of problems like mass illiteracy, poor health and lack of income and employment opportunities.

Poverty is the consequence of various factors such as illiteracy & superstition among the people, lack sufficient production infrastructure, primitive mode of agricultural production, lack of technical know-how, and lack of marketing opportunities, etc. One of the important factors for environmental problems is the rampant poverty, which make people over-dependent on the natural resource. There is two-way interlink between poverty and the environment which affect the hill ecology, *Terai* forests, misuse or underused of potential resources, and increase of the urban and industrial pollution.

The lack of good governance is also another cause for high incidence of poverty. There is an inadequate people's participation in development activities and low level of investment on human development. Such problems are compounded and can lead to multifarious problems. In the same manner, the government is falling short of effective implementation of the policies due to lack of accountability, transparency, rule of law and also the lack of political & administrative commitments. Participation of the people in the mainstream of development also holds important role for mobilising the human and other resources for development of the country. Such participation could be possible through economic, institutional, political and administrative and institutional decentralisation (Gurugharana: 1996, 31-46).

The best possible answer to these challenges could be the empowerment of the people both economically and socially by making them active and participative in the development process. Due to the infrastructure and procedural constraints including the lack of the information flow about the market opportunity, people's participation through the *free market mechanism* is limited. In the same way the decentralisation of power is limited in the papers and the local bodies still lack in resources. This has discouraged the people's participation in the *governance system* in real terms. *Participation* through the people's organisation or the NGOs could be the best means for bringing the local people in the process of development. NGOs' motivational capacity to the people and grassroots attachment, their articulation of the needs of the people, particularly of the marginalised groups is more effective than similar efforts by other sectors. An effective democracy depends upon an informed electorate and capable, responsible government. This way it can be said that NGOs, democracy and the development could be interdependent.

In view of the catalytic role of NGOs in breaking the stumbling block of poverty, the government of Nepal recognised the NGO sector as development partners. That is, NGO could both compliment and supplement the government in carrying out development activities and delivery of basic services. However, the problems facing by the NGO sector which are highlighted in the Eighth Plan are as follows:

- Policies, acts and rules to protect, promote and encourage NGOs were extremely lacking;
- The government imposed greater controls rather than allowing the NGO to run independently;
- Vague administrative procedures and lacking of co-ordination; and
- Urban concentration of NGOs (NPC: 1992, 718-719).

To overcome the above stated problems following policies were adopted during the Eighth Plan (1992-97) were as follows:

- Mobilisation of Social organisations in the field of social and economic development as they are more effective from the points of view cost, flexibility, motivation and dynamism.
- Extension of NGOs to remote and rural areas from privileged areas to perform creative and innovative works of the public importance.
- Encouragement of INGOs for running their own programs through local NGOs.
- Involving the NGO sector actively in social and economic activities at the local level in co-ordination with and under the guidance of the district development Committees, municipalities and village development committees.
- Introduction of a 'one window system' to make government decision with regard to NGO function.
- Encouragement of NGOs for empowering the weak and helpless people, classes and communities of the society to lead a life of befitting human standards on increasing the participation of women in development, on developing the appropriate technology, its transfer and use, and on conserving the environment.

- Strengthening the management capability of the NGOs in rural and remote areas through the partnership with INGOs.
- Organization of information, data and communication regarding NGOs.
- Developing effective monitoring and evaluation system (NPC: 1992, 719-721).

By adopting the policy given as above the area of partnership from the NGO sector were decided in the following activities: community and rural development, urban slums improvement, empowerment of women, improvement of environment, delivery of public health, irrigation, health education like AIDS and drug abuse, youth activities and development of moral values, including the transfer of technology. Apart from this commitment was made to develop the local/national level NGO's capabilities, simplifying the rules and regulations for the easy functioning of the NGOs, and also introduction of effective monitoring and evaluation system of the NGO works in the country (NPC: 1992, 569-572).

The NGO sector in the Ninth Plan (1997-2002) has also been taken keenly. NGOs as development partners to make the programs of NGOs in a co-ordinated manner in order to make their activities effective. Commitments have been taken for the mobilisation of NGOs in a way to make their works complementary to the development activities carried out by the government. The important contribution made by NGOs in the socio-economic development are objectively identified, and the nature, scope, resources and capabilities of such NGOs have been categorised and made co-ordinated with the local self-governance system. NGOs are encouraged to work in backward communities and especially in underdeveloped, remote regions and also to expand their activities toward those regions and communities. They are motivated to work as a facilitator vis-à-vis local institutions including District Development Committee (DDC) and Village Development Committee (VDC), educational institutions, and various community organisations and consumers (NPC: 1998, 101-102)

To achieve the objectives of NGOs as development partners following policies are set for the plan period 1997-2002:

- Improvement of policies regarding the ambiguity of Acts regarding the registration, for and working procedures,
- Involvement of NGO policy and programs for poverty-alleviation and socio-economic development,
- Development of appropriate policy and criteria for classifying the NGOs according to their area of activity and geographical region,
- Involving the NGOs in mobilisation of internal resources, training, sharing of experience,
- Mobilising INGOs in building up capability of the NGOs on the basis of their specialisation,

- Adopting a one-window system to bring about simplicity in administration to further enhance the effectiveness of resource mobilisation from the INGOs.
- Adopting institutional development of monitoring and evaluation system of NGOs activities,
- Taking special steps to honour the contributions of NGOs to a national development,
- Encouraging the competence of NGOs in building up capability and efficiency of the local bodies in accordance with the decentralisation policy.
- Making institutional arrangements to mobilise NGOs in the remote areas (NPC: 1998, 753-754).

There is much similarity in the policy contents of the Eighth and Ninth Plans. Commitments were made for facilitating and enhancing NGOs/INGOs to carry out development activities. In the Ninth Plan, long-term concept for the role of NGO operation has also been introduced. The comparative ability of NGOs is planned for using in a long-term basis for the empowerment of the people & the people's organisation and creating the conducive working environment. This can help to achieve the goal of sustainable social, economic, environmental and institutional development, and encouraging them to actively participate in the development process.

IMPLICATION OF THE NGO POLICIES ADOPTED DURING THESE PLANS PERIOD: UNEXPECTED GROWTH OF NGOS

One of the fastest growing sectors after the political change of 1990 has been the NGO sector. Registered NGOs with the concerned governmental departments were accounted for more than 16000 in 1996 (the number estimated at present is around 30,000 NGOs). (Dahal 1996, 60). However, it is difficult to get a precise number of NGOs in Nepal. Apart from this, total number of INGOs, at present, are 90 (they are also affiliated with SWC) working within the country. Out of these registered NGOs, those affiliated with Social Welfare Council (SWC) after 1992 are given in the following table:

Growth of NGOs on the basis of their functions

S.No.	Functional Area	Number of NGOs (1992)	Number of NGOs (1997)	Increased by %
1	Child Welfare	14 (2.4)	122 (2.)	871
2	Women Development	34 (5.9)	572 (9.6)	1682
3	Youth Activities	203 (35.2)	1298 (21.7)	639
4	Health Service	46 (8.0)	157 (2.6)	341
5	Education	2 (0.3)	56 (0.9)	2800
6	Service to the Blind and Handicapped	12 (2.1)	106 (1.8)	833
7	Community & Rural Development	179 (31.1)	3076 (51.4)	1718
8	Environmental Conservation	16 (2.8)	386 (6.5)	2412
9	Aids & Drug Control	6 (1.1)	28 (0.5)	466
10	Moral Development	64 (11.1)	177 (3.)	276
	Total	576 (100)	5978 (100)	1030

Figures given in the parenthesis indicate percentage Source: HMG/N National Planning Commission, EIGHTH PLAN (1992-97) p. 718 HMG/N National Planning Commission, NINTH PLAN (1997-2002) p. 700

This information reveal that Community & Rural Development Activities and Youth Activities including environment conservation and women development activities were the most preferred ones among the NGO community. However, up to early 1960s, almost 15 NGOs were registered for the delivery of health services, creation of awareness, imparting skill development training, and delivery of other social services in Nepal. In 1977, some 37 NGOs came into seen and affiliated with Social Service National Coordination Council (SNCC), a government bureau for coordinating and facilitating the NGOs. The number of affiliation has increased gently up to 220 NGOs including 52 INGOs up to 1990 (Readmaker & Tamang: 1995, 34).

Looking into the growing number of NGOs one can ask why the size of NGOs has been increasing rapidly and are they working as per the broader policy spectrum for the socio-economic transformation in the country?

The Eighth Plan for development recognizes the importance of involvement of the NGOs and the operational level. However, it does not work out the actual mandate or the strategies to involve NGOs. Thus, although there is a mushroom growth of the NGOs, due to the lack of proper guidelines there is a big confusion regarding the working relationship of the NGOs within the system (Kanchan Lama Verma: nd).

PROBLEM OF COORDINATION

In Nepal, NGOs are mostly funded by the foreign INGO/donors. Altogether 90 INGOs are working in the kingdom. Apart from this, by-lateral agencies and the local embassy also provide grants to the local NGOs. Apart from this, some ministries such as Ministry of Home, Ministry of Populations and Environment, Ministry of Health, and Ministry of Women and Social Welfare including local developmental bodies, etc. have been channeling their resources through NGOs. Priorities of investment and selection of projects often decided as per the wish of the donors and/or the concerned governmental departmental people and the role of local VDC become very much passive.

The other issue is the lack of understanding between the NGOs and the local governmental units working in the same areas. For this, some legal provision of the local bodies has been introduced; however, there is a severe lacking of co-operation among the local administrative bodies and the NGOs. A study shows the lack of proper co-ordination between the governmental and non-governmental organization which may be working with same beneficiaries for the same nature of problems but coordination may be established on the political grounds rather than developmental issues (Dhakal & Ulvila: 1999, 15-17).

There is also a problem in the transfer of resources from donor/INGOs to local NGOs in Nepal. Seeking donors'/INGOs' money is something like "hunting". Some time donors themselves create NGOs which are called DONGOs for promoting their programs (Riker: 1991, 43), however, mostly directed to implement INGOs' own interest and often make them parasite NGOs. In many cases INGOs themselves are experimenting their philosophy rather they are committed for systematic development of the country. There is also a situation of mistrust and lack of confidence between the INGOs and NGOs. Policy regarding transfer of resources from INGOs to NGOs on the basis of capacity and programs and also in a reasonable basis has not yet formulated.

CRISIS OF IMAGE

Despite NGOs are growing rapidly in Nepal, the status of NGOs themselves are in crossroads on one hand and the country also could not take much benefits from these huge number of NGO on the other hand. In other words, appropriate policies could not be adopted to make the NGOs intervention more effective to the socio-economic transformation of the country. One of the great issues that NGOs are facing is the good image in the society and good understanding with the government. With regard to the role and performance of NGO debates are going on the credibility of NGOs, type & coverage of NGO activities, and also of their working methodology

Even in the ancient period, people enjoy to involve in social works or *Paropakar* (helping others) to establish *Kirti* (eternal fame) in Nepal. '*Sewa Nai Dharma Ho'* (Service is religion) had been a common slogan among the people. But perception regarding many NGOs, at present, could not be found much positive. Ghimire presented the image of NGOs to different stakeholders like "Government officials consider NGOs to be illegal claimants to their monopoly on corruption and therefore criticize them. Business people view NGOs as fashionable, modern industries where without investment or risk high profits can be made. For the general public, social organizations are considered as another government office or a playground for the shrewd, powerful, rich urban folks. For intellectuals, they are no more than begging bowls" Ghimire: (ND.), 17).

It is said that many NGOs activists are not for delivery of service to the targeted beneficiaries but are taking services in the name of service delivery. These type of NGOs according to Bhattachan are termed as 'Pajero NGOs', 'Briefcase NGOs', Suitcase NGOs, 'Green Dollars NGOs', 'Family NGOs' etc (Bhattachan: 1998,15). There is a common to see a luxurious life style from among bigger NGO people. The government of Nepal has a policy for facilitating NGOs by giving subsidy facilities, however, there is a lacking of the policy to controlling the misuse of such subsidies.

Ultimately, these all jeopardize the *accountability* of the NGOs. Accountability can be described as 'mechanisms by which the agencies concerned can be held responsible for their actions and whether they fulfill the agreements and conditions they enter into, including adherence to the values and principles for which they stand' (Edwards and Hulme 1996). However, it is very difficult to measure the accountability of any organization. The government through its policy measures could make NGOs accountable to the concerned stakeholders for getting relief from such blames.

CENTRALIZE- DECENTRALIZATION

In Nepal, almost 89 percent of the people reside in the village. The socio-economic condition of the people in the rural areas is much more vulnerable than of the urban centres. One can assume NGOs reach to the grassroots where the government may not. But the most of the NGOs are located in the urban centres particularly in Kathmandu and also in other parts of the urban centres for making money. For this, these urban based NGOs often cry for grants and aid and secure from peddling Nepal's poverty and helplessness (The Rising Nepal: 1997, 4). Even the government agency like SWC has also been supporting urban-based NGOs more than the NGOs working in the rural areas. Following Table gives an example of urban concentration of the SWC.

District-wise Institutional Development Fund

Rank for getting SWC Grants	1995/96 District No.of NGO Amount	1997/98 District No.of NGO Amount	1997/98 District No.of NGO Amount
First	Kathmandu 31 Rs. 15,10,800	Kathmandu 25 Rs. 22,61,410	Kathmandu 100 Rs. 13,20,000
Second	Rupandehi 15 Rs. 8,35,000.	Dhanusha 10 Rs. 9,68,805	Sarlahi 18 Rs. 5,70,000.
Third	Dhanusha 15 Rs. 7,26,500.	Sarlahi 4 Rs. 4,00,000.	Dhanusha 20 Rs. 3,00,000.
Others	Others 84 Rs. 43,24,800	Others 33 Rs. 28,15320	Others 265 33,70,000.
Total	73,97,100 145	64,45,535 72	55,60,000 403

Source: **SWC News** Aug./Sep.1998 and **Samajik Sewa Samachar** Jestha/Asar 2055 and Kartik 2055

During the study period the NGOs based in the urban centers like Kathmandu, Rupandehi, Dhanusha and Sarlahi got around half of the total resources delivered to the NGOs. The policy commitment regarding the promotion of NGOs of the rural sector seems silent.

In many cases NGOs are much more· happy only for demonstration and easy work rather than actual service delivery or involving in the development work for the social change. Many NGOs were found concentrated at the capital and doing seminars at Five Stars hotels for making very attractive reports to submit to the donors and also to the concerned governmental departments. Former Prime Minister G.P. Koirala in one inaugural meeting of the NGOs said, "…it would be better for NGOs to spend their resources on a drinking water system in a village than in such talkshops." (Rademacher & Tamang: 1995, 37). This indicates that the volume of talk is more than the volume of work from the NGOs.

QUESTION OF TRANSPARENCY

The other burning issue of the NGOs is the transparency of their source and volume of resources and sometimes types of works. Questions regarding transparency and accountability have been raising from the streets to the parliamentary sessions including other public forums. The annual estimated development grants channeled through the NGOs could be NPR. 5 to 6 billion (Equivalent to US $ 88,75,740). However, NGOs are rather concentrating on paper work and are alone defining and classifying their work instead of producing the results that serve the target people in a transparent way. (The Kathmandu Post 1998, 1).

In 1999, the government enforces a rule regarding NGO performance specially keeping transparency. According to this provision the NGOs should be registered initially and renewed annually to be eligible for acquiring grants especially foreign money. They should also furnish their audit report, progress report, source and amount of funding. The ultimate objective of this provision is "transparency". NGOs and their federation became impatient and hostile, for example, when Kathmandu and Lalitpure district administration offices denied renewing some NGOs. (The Kathmandu Post, Feb 18,1999; The Rising Nepal, Feb. 18,1999; Aajako Samachar Patra (National dailly), Feb. 18, 1999).

It might be true that many registered (sometime not) NGOs have been taking money and disappearing from the seen. David classified such NGOs as "COME'N GOs". This means that there are paper organizations that never operated or operate only one project, and then disintegrated. They see funding as a lucrative opportunity and package large and expensive proposals for donors. (David: 1993, 137.138). The government should develop effective policy that could be effective to control such anomalies.

LACK OF MONITORING AND EVALUATION

Policies regarding monitoring and evaluation of the NGO performance has been lacking, however, policy commitments stated in the Ninth Plan (1997-2002) can be taken as a positive step in this regard. The responsibility of evaluation and monitoring the NGO activities is bestowed on SWC. SWC is equipped with some 100 manpower which is naturally insufficient to monitor and SWC affiliated 8000 NGOs and 90 INGOs on one hand and on the other the frequent change of the SWC executive members particularly the Member-Secretary (executive head) SWC failing to monitor and evaluate the NGOs working in the country. INGOs/dorors, which fund for local NGOs are also not able to monitor the use and/or misuse of such development cooperation. Therefore one should rely on the reports prepared by the concerned NGOs.

CONCLUSIONS

NGOs should be founded on the principle of accountability, networking, co-ordinating and vertical integration, advocacy and campaign, empowerment, capacity building, access, relief, and management and implementation of the program. Apart from this, NGOs have been a good mechanism for the transfer of the foreign resources and also mobilising the local resources. NGOs are expected to penetrate the grassroots and motivate for the empowerment activities. For this, the government has adopted in its national policy for involving NGOs as development partners particularly since the Eighth Plan (1992-97). As a result the functional and numerical growth of NGOs has been witnessed in Nepal. However, there has been some discrepancy between the content and spirit of policy and the implementation practices of NGO in Nepal. It requires more commitments from all the stakeholders – the government, NGO communities, and the people at large for the effective use of NGOs expertise towards the socio-economic enhancement of the country.

REFERENCES

Aajako Samachar Patra (National dailly), Year 4, No. 39 Feb. 18, 1999

Anheier, Helmut K. & Seibel, Wolfgang (Eds. 1990): *The Third Sector. Comparative Studies of Non-profit Organisations*, Berlin: Walter de Gruyter.

Bhattachan Krishna Bahadur (1998:0 "NGO & INGO in Nepal: Reality and Bhram"(in Nepali), *Bikas* (Quarterly) Vol. 7, No. 11. Kathmandu: Atmanirvar Bikas Manch.

Burkey Stan (1993): *PEOPLE FIRST A Guide to self-reliant, Participatory Rural Development*: London: Zed Books Ltd.

Brown, L. David and David C. Korten, 1991: "Working More Effectively with Non-governmental Organisations" in *Paul and Israel*, 1991.

CECI (1992): The Potentials of Nepali NGOs. Vol. 1. Kathmandu: Canadian Centre for International Studies and Co-operation.

Chand, Diwakar (1991): *Development through Non-Governmental Organisations in Nepal*: Kathmandu: Institute for National Development Research and Social Services (INDRASS).

Chand, Diwakar (1998): " The Role of Civil Society in Democratisation NGO perspective" in Shrestha, Anand (ed.), *The Role of Civil Society and Democratisation in Nepal*: Kathmandu: NEFAS.

Clark John (1991): *Democratising Development: The Role of Voluntary Organisations*, Connecticut: Kumarian Press.

Dhakal, Tek Nath & Ulvila, Marko (March 1999): *Institutional Analysis of Markhu VDC with Emphasis on Non-Governmental Organisation* (An unpublished Report on NGOs in Development Research Project Vorking Document 3).

Edwards, Michael (1994): 'NGOs in the Age of Information' *IDS Bulletin* Vol. 25, No. 2

Edwards, M. and D. Hulme: 1996: *Beyond the Magic Bullet: NGO Performance and Accountability in the Post-Cold War World*: West Hartfort, CT: Kumarian Press.

Esman, Milton J. and Uphoff, Norman: 1984: Local *Orgnaizations, Intermediaries in Rural Development*. Ithaca, New Yourk: Rural Development committee, Cornell University.

Fisher, William F., 1997: "Doing Good? The Politics and Antipolitics of NGO Practices" *Annual Review of Anthropology.*

Guru-Gharana, Kishor Kumar (April 1996): "Development Strategy for Nepal Perception from Below" in Dahal Dev Raj & Guru-Gharana Kishor Kumar (eds.): *Development Strategy for Nepal.* Kathmandu: Nepal Foundation for Advanced Studies.

Guru-gharana, Kishor Kumar, nd.: "Poverty Alleviation issues" In *Social development in Nepal.* UNAN: Kathmandu: 83.

Ghimire, Jagadish, Acharya, Narhari, et.al: (ND.): NGO Policy of Nepal: A Study: Kathmandu: NGO Federation of Nepal: In Rademacher, Anne & Tamang, Deepak (1995): *Democracy Development & NGOs: Kathmandu:* SEARCH: pp.32-33.

HMG/N (1992): *Village Development Act 1992,* Kathmandu: Ministry of Local Development.

HMG/N (1992): *Municipality Act 1992,* Kathmandu, and Ministry of Local Development.

HMG/N (1992): *District Development Act 1992,* Kathmandu, and Ministry of Local Development.

HMG/N (1977): *Social Service Act 1977,* Kathmandu: Ministry of Law & Justice.

HMG/N (1992): *Social Welfare Act 1992,* Kathmandu: Ministry of Labour and Social Welfare.

Hulme, David (N.D.) Social Development Research and the Third Sector. NGOs as Users and Subjects of Social Inquiry, in: Booth, David (Ed.). *Rethinking Social Development. Theory, Research & Practice.* Essex: Longman. P. 251-275.

IDS (1985): *Non-governmental institutions and Process for Development in Nepal,* Kathmandu: IDS

James, E., 1990:'Economic Theories of the Nonprofit Sector', in *Anheier and Seibel,* 1990: 21-31.

Korten David C. (1990): *Getting to the 21st Century: Voluntary Action and the Global Agenda.* Connetticut: Kumarian Press.

Kanchan Lama Verma: nd, "Social Integration Issues" in *Social Development in Nepal.* UNAN: p. 122.

Lama et.al, (January 1992): "Non-Governmental Organisations and Grassroots Development" in *Administration and Management Review:* Number 6: Lalitpur: NASC.

Mario, Pardon (Autumn 1987): "Non-Government Development Organisations: From Development Aid to Development Co-operation" *World Development,* Vol. 15.

Nepal South Asia Centre (1998): *Nepal Human Development Report 1998.* Kathmandu: Nepal South Asia Centre.

NPC, HMG/N (1992): *The Eighth Plan (1992-1997),* Kathmandu, and National

Planning Commission.

NPC, HMG/N (1997): *APPROACH PAPER of the Ninth Plan (1997 – 2002)*, Kathmandu, National Planning Commission.

NPC, HMG/N (1998): *NINTH PLAN (1997-2002)*: Kathmandu: National Planning Commission.

OECD (1988): *Voluntary Aid for Development: The Role of Non-Government Organisation*. Paris: OECD.

Philip Elridge (1988): "Non-Government Organisation and the Role of the State in Indonesia." A Paper presented to conference on State and Civil Society in Indonesia, Monash University, in Salauddin Aminuzzaman *Development Management and The Role of NGOs in Bangladesh, Administrative Change*, Vol. XXIV, No. 1 (July December 1996).

Private Agencies Collaborating Together (PACT) (1987): *The Non-governmental Organisations Sector of Nepal: A Study*: Kathmandu: Prepared by PACT Team for USAID.

Rademacher and Tamang, Deepek (1995): *Democracy, Development and NGOs*, Kathmandu: SEARCH.

Riker, James V. 1991: *Contending Perspectives for Interpreting Government NGO relations in South and South East Asia: Constrains, Challenges, and the search for common ground in Rural Development*. Background paper prepared for the APDC Regional Dialogue GO-NGO relations in Asia: Prospects and challenges for improving the Policy Environment for people centred Development: March 11-15, 1991. Chiengmai, Thailand, Malaysia: APDC. Quoted in Maskay, Bishwa Keshar (1998): *Non-Governmental Organizations In Development Search for a new Vision*, Kathmandu: Centre for Development and Governance.

SWC (1997): *Samajik Sewa Samachar*: Year 10, Vol. 1 Shrawan-Aswin, 2054: Kathmandu: SWC.

SWC (1998): *SWC News* August-September 1998: Kathmandu: SWC.

SWC (1998): *Samajik Sewa Samachar*: Jestha-Ashar 2055: Kathmandu: SWC.

SWC (1998): *Samajik Sewa Samachar*: Kartik 2055: Kathmandu: SWC.

The Kathmandu Post, (August 1, 1998): "Monitor NGOs properly, say MPs" Vol. VI, No. 163.

The Kathmandu Post Vol. VI No. 356, Feb 18,1999 Kathmandu

The Rising Nepal (National Daily), (Dec. 23, 1997), Kathmandu, Nepal

The Rising Nepal Vol. XXXIV, No 65 Feb. 18,1999).

Tuladhar, Jyoti (1991): *"The Growth and Development of NGOs in the 1990s"* a seminar paper presented in "National NGO Conference" Kathmandu, Sept. 23-25, 1991.

Tvedt, Terje (1998): NGOs' Role at 'The End of History': Norwegian Policy and the New Paradigm. In: Farhad & Myllyla, Susanna (Eds. 1998): *NGOs Under Challenge: Dynamics and Drawbacks in Development*. Helsinki: Ministry for Foreign Affairs of Finland, Department for International Development Co-operation. P. 63-83.

UNDP (1997): *Human Development Report*: Oxford University Press.

Uphoff, Norman and Cohen, J., *Feasibility and Application for Rural Development: Analysis of Asian Experience* Ithaca, New York: Rural Development committee, Cornell University.

Weisbrod, B.A., 1988, The Nonprofit Economy, Cambrige, MA: Harvard University Press: Quoted in Terje Tvedt, 1998: *Angels of Mercy or Development Diplomats?* Africa World Press: Trenton, p. 41.

9. DEVELOPMENT CONTRADICTION AND EXPECTATIONS FROM NGOS

Dipak Gyawali

There are certain words that symbolise and legitimise an age, and development is one such term. With the end of the Second World War, overt imperialism could not be justified but the need for neo-colonialist resource extraction from the Periphery to the Centre was an imperative as ingrained in the new world order as in the old. Development became the new "White Man's Burden" that legitimised economic intervention, as development aid, both in the Centre and the Periphery. However, since the collapse of the Second World towards the end of the 1980s, there was little by way of geopolitical imperative for the First World to continue appeasing the elite of the Third World. Furthermore, examination of the after-effects of development by egalitarian activists is showing that one man's development can often be another man's degradation. As a result, the last half of the 20th Century, which may even be termed the Age of Development and more specifically the age of Foreign Aid, is now coming to an end.

One early sign of this age coming to an end lay in the shift of Western donors from funding Third World governments to funding NGOs. By the mid-1980s, with the failure of various development decades from drinking water to health through the state mechanism, donors had come to realise the rent-seeking character of most Third World bureaucracies that were far removed from the ideals of civil service. What was difficult to justify, in front of the critical press and civil society in the North, was the tax "paid by the poor in the rich countries to the rich in the poor countries" in the name of development aid. Hence the attractiveness of the idea of channelling "charity" efforts such as grants and poverty alleviation programs through international NGOs and their local counterparts. Compared to the previous arrangement of such financial resources flowing to sovereign governments with prickly diplomatic sensitivities, this new arrangement had, for Northern fund managers, the advantage of easier accountability on demand and a dependency structure in their favour.

One important factor in the rural areas of the Third World is that the informal economy dominates. In other words, an overwhelming majority of the population of the Third World is outside of the formalised "national economy" in which it is either unable to participate or can participate only under unequal and demeaning terms. Southern population can be divided into "omnivores" versus "ecosystem people" and "eco-refugees" depending on how they are able to capture global resources (Gadgil and Guha, 1995). Omnivores are those rich in the South whose resource catchment is the entire planet (no different from the Northern rich). The others, the ecosystem people, form the bulk of what is

known as the informal world, and either live in the villages where mo
needs come from within a few tens of kilometres of their homes
margins of islands of prosperity such as the slums of overcrowded citie
the population of the latter is more than 80% while that of the former is less than
20%.

There have been several attempts to define the informal world. One way is
to distinguish between property rights protected by the formal legal system and
informal property rights protected by self-policed contracts. By this count,
informal economy would account for perhaps up to 70% of a country's gross
national product. Another way of looking at the informal economy has been to
distinguish between goods and services that are marketed but escape
enumeration, regulation or other type of public monitoring or auditing. Other
authors further distinguish informally marketed goods and services that escape
enumeration into legal and illegal goods and services, implying that the informal
is not illegal but one where the reach of the state and its vision is absent. It is a
world inhabited by the vulnerable and the marginalised. What these definitions
do is to reconstitute the boundary of our understanding of economic activities to
include the vast reality of coping with everyday living that the majority of the
population in South Asia indulges in, but which have yet to see academic insight,
policy foresight or legal hindsight (Gyawali, 1997b).

Much of natural resource management in the South falls under the purview
of the informal. This is true as much of forests as of irrigation. In Nepal, of the
roughly half a million hectares of irrigated land, the informal and traditional
farmer-managed irrigation systems account for almost 80% whereas
government-managed systems (supported by all the foreign aid for the last forty
years) accounts for about 20%. Forests in Nepal, especially in the vicinity of
hamlets in the hills, were under the purview of the informal. In the name of
accelerating development, they were nationalised in 1957 with disastrous
consequences to the common property. In the last decade, the mistake has been
rectified slowly and they are being handed back to the communities through the
community forestry program. Another good example is the private housing
sector in Nepal: informal contractors conduct almost all the activity in this area.

Where the state has no capacity to influence the vast set of economic
activities of the poor in the informal sector, neither would foreign aid agencies.
Hence the flight to NGOs. However, in opting for this path, there are pitfalls as
well as the case below illustrates.

CASE OF A NEPALI NGO SWABALAMBAN

To illustrate the dynamics of the shifting roles of the government and the NGOs
in the informal sector, an account of a Nepali NGO Swabalamban and its
successor, Rural Self-reliance Development Center (RSDC) is given below.

The concept of Swabalamban (or sustainable development of the poor by the poor") was started by an ex-finance secretary in February 1985, in part due to the frustrations of failed development from the conventional methods of interventions. Nepal had seen a lot of development efforts by foreign aid agencies since the end of the Second World War, starting with Harry Truman's Point Four program. One of the early entrants were the Swiss who continue to be involved in Nepal's rural development. Swabalamban was started with an initial funding of US$ 2000 from the Swiss INGO Helvetas at a time when "integrated rural development" concepts were in vogue. The year 1985 was also the year when the conditionalities of "structural adjustment program" placed Nepal government under the tutelage of the World Bank and IMF by opening up several of its closed sectors to market interventions.

In the initial days, the concepts of Swabalamban were vague. Beyond the recognition that conventional development approaches had failed to reach the poor, that a new approach was needed which could not be a state agency-led affair, there was no "model" as such. It evolved in the years of intensive grassroots work in the villages of Palpa in the mid-hills of mid-western Nepal. The first task was to give the poor the confidence that their lot could be better if they took the initiative for change in their own hands. Towards this end, a Swabalamban motivator stayed in the village with the poor for at least six months working with them and inculcating in them the confidence they were lacking. The simple equation of capital accumulation (increase income - decrease useless consumption) was translated into strict curtailment of wealth-frittering activities such as drinking, gambling and ostentatious festivals. These had become the traditional structural means of assuring that people stayed in poverty.

The next task was to increase income. The people had the skills, especially among the dalits such as the blacksmiths, but were in bonded generational debt and were severely short of capital. Though the capital requirement was minimal by urban standards, it was still unavailable. The method used by the motivators was to set up an "income generating group" or IGG where the integrity of bond between the poor themselves acted as the collateral for the loan given to the group. The first loan of Rs 2700 to an IGG of 6 blacksmiths. They used Rs 2100 to buy copper sheets from which they made vessels and utensils. These were sold in the market for Rs 2920 and, after deducting labour costs, a profit of Rs 460 was made by the IGG. (RSDC, 1998). In this manner, a poverty alleviation program "of the poor by the poor" was born.

Even though IGGs and micro-credits for income generation (a term that became fashionable almost ten years later) became important activities of Swabalamban, it was not its main goal. The primary purpose was still awareness building, inculcating self-confidence in the poor that they themselves can improve their lot, and using organisation for such empowerment. As a small example, before a loan is given, the person receiving it has to learn to sign his or her name and not just place a thumbprint. The idea is not to claim non-existent literacy but to give the person a sense of self-esteem, and it has worked almost like magic.

The early problems of Swabalamban were related to the reactions from the feudal elements of society who were displeased with the way their bonded labourers were escaping from their grip. Swabalamban had an anti-Panchayat, anti-feudal and anti-bureaucratic thrust. This also earned it the wrath of these political elements who saw Swabalamban as an undesirable subversive activity, which led to official harassment. Despite this, the program grew popular and expansion was by way of mimesis in adjoining villages. However, after the collapse of the Panchayat system in April 1990 and the restoration of multi-party democracy, Swabalamban activities expanded rapidly. It had been started in 1985 as an "action research" program within an institutional set-up that did not reflect the voluntarism of Swabalamban (it was within a "consultancy"). The inherent tension between the functionaries of the consultancy and Swabalamban resulted in the motivators of Swabalamban leaving the organisation to set up to set up their own Rural Self-reliance Development Center.

With these changes, the activities of RSDC expanded rapidly, eventually covering 26 village administrative units (VDCs) in 14 out of 75 districts of Nepal. Some of the work in places like remote north Gorkha was about seven walking days from the nearest road head, where Swabalamban motivators were the first "bikasey manchhe" (or development people) to come to these villages even as government employees had never reached them in recent times. Some of the notable successes of RSDC related to capital accumulation in making IGGs self-reliant and taking their members out of the bonded labour trap. There was tremendous growth in awareness, especially among women groups where women who would otherwise have stayed behind purdah were taking active part in public meetings and demanding their rights. Development works such as water supply or vegetable growing were much cheaper and better maintained than similar work done by government agencies. Most important, there was a sense of voluntarism among IGG members that contributed to the development of social capital.

Swabalamban then began to face a new set of challenges. First, the concept of "social mobilisation" was taken up by other newly formed NGOs, so RSDC was no longer either the sole activist/service provider or the most professionally streamlined. Second, and most important, there were other donor agencies such as the German GTZ who became involved more deeply, bringing their concept of what swabalamban was. In essence, there was a fight between seeing Swabalamban as a force for empowerment and social mobilisation or an efficient "delivery agent" for donor agencies.

The matters came to a head towards May 1996 when attempts to correct the tilt in favour of empowerment as against delivery of services led to friction with the GTZ. Of the two major supporters of RSDC, the GTZ was already

ing 60% of the funding and Helvetas and DANIDA about 40%. There
sure on RSDC to take up the job of mobilising local people for building
re called "green roads". There was also the problem of incentive grants
had a poor accountability structure to the RSDC board, it being mostly
within the purview of the donor agency program officer and the RSDC executive
director. The attempt to bring some transparency in this activity brought about
the first conflict between the board and the donor agency, which managed to
engineer a split within RSDC, taking a chunk of motivators to form a new
organisation that was more pliable to implementing its plans. RSDC continued
under a new management, but it too is hamstrung by the fact that it is dependent
on western donors for funding, albeit, its sources are more diversified.

NGOs AND ME POWER STRUCTURE

Because the evolution of the nation-state has been different in Western Europe
and in the South, nationalism in the South has become one of the major tactics
for organising the majority of the people for reproducing state power, in the
process alienating the vast collage of minorities (Ahmed, 1996). The impact of
this process has been the growth of a "security state" where the security
apparatus is increasingly used against diversity-seeking minorities. Another
consequence has been the hijacking of Development to benefit the class of
omnivores.

This alienation of the state from the masses in the South has led to the
failure of Development. After four decades of development aid, the net flow of
resources is from the South to the North and not the other way around, it being
the bottom-line indicator of its failure. While Development doctors diagnose ills
in Southern societies for this failure (conjuring up such terms as "low absorptive
capacity", "weak institutional base" etc. and essentially blaming the victims of
Development), foreign aid has become addictive to the state structures of the
South even when there are signs of increasing aid fatigue in the North. The gap
between the intended and actual beneficiaries, between intent and performance,
is too wide to be ignored.

To enforce the Omnivore's definition of Development - with which an
increasingly clamorous set of voices is not in consonance - the repressive power
of the state is used with increasing frequency. Large water resources projects are
good examples of such misuse (Gyawali, 1997a & 1998). In India, such projects
have displaced twenty million people, some of them multiple times with
negligible compensation for their trouble. The question - whose Development? -
becomes quite relevant since this is the Development of the Omnivores against
the others. This Globalization of Development has been carried out by using the
State as its beast of burden, which bears the ultimate brunt of sovereign loans and
the concomitant covenants. Essentially for the poor, this alienation from the
State has also meant that it is increasingly being perceived not as a

confidence-inspiring institutional resource for enhancing their security but a danger full of rapacity.

ROLE OF VOLUNTARISM

A way of perceiving the role of foreign aid in development is shown in Figure 1. Basic active institutional forces at work in any society can be classified into three groups: the State, the Market and the Civil Society (Douglas, 1992).

Under ideal conditions, the State would be characterised by attributes such as rule of law, an equitable and just taxation system as well as a transparent exercise of power. Similarly, the Market would be competitive, with sufficient players, equal information among them and without any bias or favouritism towards any one of them. Civil Society would also be genuine wherein there would be modesty in their lifestyles and living, strong voluntary ethics, diversity in trusteeship, and fiscal transparency. A harmonious balance between these three forces would contribute to a society's innovative creativity (through the Market), just and equitable regulation (through the State) and timely caution and upholding of values other than profit (through an alert Civil Society). It would be a contested but civilised terrain (Thompson & Gyawali, 1997).

Much of the South finds itself far away from this ideal. Essentially it has become an uncontested terrain in the institutional sense, and Development Aid has to shoulder much of the blame for it. While the nation-state had never acquired the same overwhelming powers that it did in Bismarkian Europe, the Bretton Woods arrangement and the allied "united nations" concept conferred upon Southern nation-states *zamindari* rights over its citizens and spaces. It allowed governments the rights to play with the future through sovereign loans. For a feudal state apparatus, this boon was god-sent. Foreign Aid became akin to nutrient inflow in a pond resulting in *eutrophic algal* bloom: government agencies soon began to take over village and community functions, from resource management to small-scale business. Aided and abetted by Foreign Aid, governments became businessmen and monopolised social service.

Markets in such an uncontested terrain became distorted or phantom markets. In place of a level playing field, one began to see monopolies, exchange rate controls and multiple rates favouring cronies, as well as a License Raj of tariffs, quotas and permits that allow a rent-seeking feudocracy to extract surplus at various stages of the Development game. Extreme examples of state overtaking the functions of the market are the classic despots of Congo and Philippines.

Civil Society too turned phantom when the social sector lost its voluntariness as it became Developmentalised. In many Southern states, the governments monopolised social service and prevented independent voluntary associations to function. NGOs became fronts for business or politics, and are known by various descriptive acronyms: GONGOS (government-organised

NGOs), DONGOS (donor-organised NGOs), or business-organised NGOs (BONGOs) etc. In extreme cases, a donor-funded and backed NGO (Taliban in Afganistan) became the state. These contradictions are illustrated in the annexed figure 'Order and Disjunctions'.

TO TAKE OR NOT TO TAKE?

In the post-Cold War 1 990s, with the outbreak of Democracy in many Southern countries, the uncontested terrain enjoyed by the state began to be challenged. In reaction, those who advocated state-led Development now are beginning to argue for a market-led path. While global governance at the State level was the norm since the end of the Second World War, economic liberalisation favouring the free play of multi-national corporations is being propagated as the new mantra of salvation. As our diagram indicates, a two-legged stool is no more stable than a one-legged one. What is missing, as the third leg is global Civil Society that is motivated by concerns other than the market's concern for profit and the state's proclivity for control. The question here is of the degree of voluntariness as opposed to urges for profit or control.

There are several challenges before secular voluntarism in our midst. First, the most talked about question is whether voluntary organisations should take foreign funding or not. Unquestioningly taking funding would easily convert a voluntary activist organisation into an efficient "delivery agent" of western donor agencies as the above case shows. On the other hand, staying away from these global resources would deprive the volunteers of effective means to further their cause. The question probably lies in the manner in which the funds are availed of, under what conditions and what structure of accountability. The other problem lies in the growing politicisation of NGOs that function as fronts for political parties. In such a scenario, there would be a crisis of confidence and ultimately a negative image of voluntary organisations.

In bringing about true voluntariness, the real challenge is to find out how globalisation of civil society concerns can occur. It is easy for multi-national companies to talk of global markets and the international association of state bureaucracies to promulgate global protocols and treaties. It is much more difficult for global action among local activist groups whose arena is necessarily at the grassroots. But the need is there if global rapacity and international bureaucratic stultification is to be kept at bay. It is also needed to keep voluntary societies truly voluntary.

REFERENCES

Ahmed, I., 1996: *A Post-Nationalist South Asia*, Himal vol. 9 no. 5, Kathmandu.

Douglas, M., 1992: *Risk and Blame: Essays in Cultural Theory*; Routledge, London.

Gadgil, M. and Guha, R. 1995: *Ecology and Equity: The Use and Abuse of Nature in Contemporary India*; Routledge and Penguin Books India (P) Ltd.

Gyawali, D., 1998: *Patna, Delhi and Environmental Activism: Institutional Forces behind Water Conflict in Bihar*, WATER NEPAL, vol. 6 no. 1, Kathmandu.

Gyawali, D., 1997a: *Foreign Aid and the Erosion of Local Institutions: An Autopsy of Arun3 from Inception to Abortion*; in C. Thomas and P. Wilkin (ed) Globalization and the South, Macmillan London and St. Martin's Press New York.

Gyawali, D., 1997b: *Economic Security in a Predominantly Informal World: South Asian Realities and Global Elation with Privatization*; in Iftekharuzzaman (ed) Regional Economic Trends and South Asian Security, Regional Center for Strategic Studies Colombo and Manohar Publishers Delhi.

RSDC, 1998 Bipannata Bata Mukti Ka Lagi Swabalamban (in Nepali: Swabalamban for Liberation from Poverty), Rural Self-Reliance Development Center, Kathmandu.

Nandy, A., 1996: *Nation, State and Self-Hatred*; Himal, vol. 9 no. 5, Kathmandu.

Thompson, M. and Gyawali, D., 1997: *Transboundary Risk Management in the South: A Comparative Example from the Himalaya*; LOS-Senteret Notat 9721, Norwegian Research Centre in Organisation and Management, Bergen.

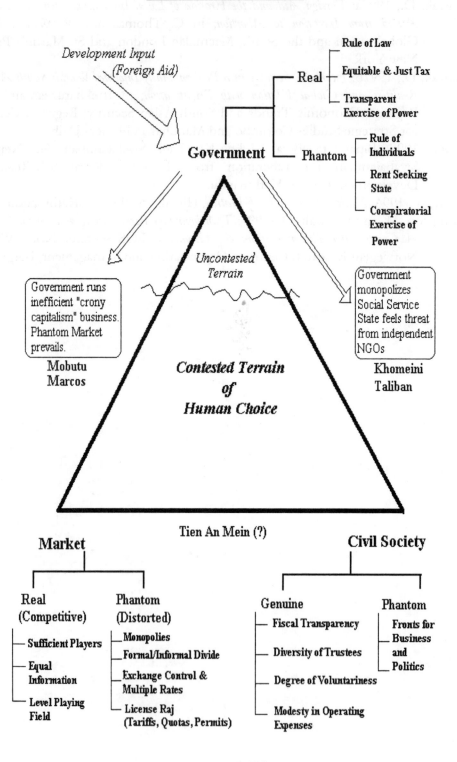

D. Gyawali/Helsinki/9.98

<u>_Order and Disjunctions_</u>

Development Input
(Foreign Aid)

Government

Real
— Rule of Law
— Equitable & Just Tax
— Transparent Exercise of Power

Phantom
— Rule of Individuals
— Rent Seeking State
— Conspiratorial Exercise of Power

Uncontested Terrain

Government runs inefficient "crony capitalism" business. Phantom Market prevails.

Mobutu
Marcos

Government monopolizes Social Service State feels threat from independent NGOs

Khomeini
Taliban

Contested Terrain
_of_
Human Choice

Tien An Mein (?)

Market

Real (Competitive)
— Sufficient Players
— Equal Information
— Level Playing Field

Phantom (Distorted)
— Monopolies
— Formal/Informal Divide
— Exchange Control & Multiple Rates
— License Raj (Tariffs, Quotas, Permits)

Civil Society

Genuine
— Fiscal Transparency
— Diversity of Trustees
— Degree of Voluntariness
— Modesty in Operating Expenses

Phantom
— Fronts for Business and Politics

10. FOUNDATION OF AN AUTONOMOUS CIVIL SOCIETY AND THE ENVIRONMENT OF THE CITIZENS IN NEPAL

Govind P. Dhakal

BACKGROUND

Democratisation, citizen participation, human rights and the code of conduct in administration are the fundamental things that have won the world interest in administrative theories and practices in the wave of democratisation. Unlike old practices where traditional administration and military dictators were regularised as agents of change and modernisation, the present practices are valued for the masterpiece of civil society based on the principles of peoples' participation democratically in the process of socio-economic development of the society. The overall development of the people is not possible in isolation as was conceived by Max Weber in his theorisation of bureaucratic principles in administration but is possible only through democratic decentralisation with the growing number of autonomous people's organisations based on the socio-economic, political and religio-cultural background. The foundation of an autonomous civil society is enabled and supported only when the administration has a limited role to play . The limited role of the administration and the empowerment of the citizens through well established socio-economic structures or a liberalised economic structures in often seen and realised in advanced and developed political economy than in an underdevelopment one.

Sometimes, there appears a tension between unfolding a democratic civil society and the traditional economic structure. However, the civil society can impact on the economic fabric favourably in economic change. This, in turn, may lead to a stronger and firmly rooted civil society which may enable the structures to act in a better way.   The very concept of bureaucracy-led development is no longer valid as it has proved to be counter productive by alienating the poor, down trodden and marginalised people for whom development is primarily meant (Bava 1997, 5). Since the 1980s there has been a policy shift in development due to the economic liberalisation and the weakening of the policy of development through commanding, centralised and bureaucratic planning and development.

Voluntary or Non-Governmental organisations (NGOs) have, in this scenario, emerged as an alternative to bureaucracy and state controlled agencies for achieving development. Peoples' participation has come to be accepted as an essential condition of good governance and a democratic civil society. NGOs, in this regard, have come to help achieve the goal of good governance and empowerment of the citizens. Now the recognition of NGOs as citizen's organisation believed to bring about community development by harnessing local peoples' participation, initiatives and resources. Although there are some dilemmas in the activities of NGOs i.e. in involving voluntary association in development, these may be counted as reform vs. revolution, autonomy vs. accountability, violence vs. non-violence, youth vs. aged and direct action vs. law.

AUTONOMOUS SOCIETY: A BIRDS EYE VIEW

The crux of democracy consists in its social organisation and social base (Kothari 1987, 438). The key democratic polity is a basic concept of a social and political infrastructure as much as the economy does. Without infrastructure we would be reduced to a mechanical solidarity in place of an organic solidarity. To make a democracy functioning effectively there has to be a lot of organisations sensitive to the needs of the people and to be rooted in the racial structures. These social structures are formed variety of ways. Even for making electoral democracy effective we need voluntary agencies that are formed on the spirit of voluntarism and not agencies for external bodies organisations and quasi-organisations constituted on specific goals of their members and draw their resources not for the survival of their group. Such organisations can exist only if they are supported by economic agents which draw their own resources form activities that do not depend on the state and which are exchanged in the market. Drawing resources through the governmental institutional set up goes against autonomy. However, autonomy does not mean only autonomy of economic activities but also mean to non-economic activities like human rights protection, preservation of environmental activities, and the like. These also sometimes, have to be depended heavily on the economic actors to run their activities. (see e.g. Elsenhans 1997)

The autonomy cannot be realised unless a competitive society -- free from state protection is built. Also autonomy does not mean anything unless grass-root level person or a marginal society is well addressed to be empowered. People in the professional pursuit often argue that the technical progress and economic efficiency lead toward achieving this autonomy. They, however forget that technological progress may lead to luxuries to certain section and economic efficiency may be a cause to more surplus to the already advantaged. Therefore, mutual benefit and trust among social and political process is a pre-condition for a durable arrangement for an autonomous society. The drive to democratisation and increasing self-organisation, are achieved through investment either by state or private sectors to empower poor or through programmes aiming to assist the poor so that they can increase their purchasing power (ibid., 11).

Governance, a highly fashioned and rhetoric in the question of development management, has to strive for local capacity building so that development becomes self sustaining. The local capacity building is responsible only when (Dahal 1996, 7):

- • - Specific managerial and professional skill development is done;
- • - A training task is carried on;
- • - The public service is reformed in consonance with the need of decentralised development;
- • - Private sectors are encouraged to enhance all sectors development;
- • - Popular participation to pursue the national goals; and
- • - Existence of national development culture.

The governance applies to the power in a variety of institutional context. The object of which is to direct control and regulate activities in the interest of people as citizens, voters and workers (Robinson 1996, 347). UNDP identifies some key features of good governance in a civil society which include (UNDP 1995, 22):

- • - Political accountability and legitimacy;
- • - A fair and reliable judicial service system;
- • - Bureaucratic accountability;
- • - Freedom of information and freedom of expression;
- • - Effective and efficient public sector management and co-operation with
- • civil society organisations;
- • - Decentralising Power for Autonomy of Civil Societies

The quest for the foundation of an autonomous civil society can only be realised when centralised power and authority is well decentralised to the development actors in various forms. This is one if the means available before us for enlarging the influence of those who are ready to mobilise resources other than the voting politics. Also ensures a sort of autonomous co-existence where actors are equalised in respect of their difference of opinion. The decentralisation of power and development of autonomous civil society has been a long felt need due to inflexibility, slow moving, non-responsive and non-pragmatic behaviour of public bureaucracy and profit seeking nature of public organisations. In course of searching best alternative to development partners the international organisations and donor agencies have started to rely more and more on the newly recognised alternative or third sector organisations (Mälkiä & Hossain 1998, 22). The assumption is that the third sectors activities would promote to reach more effectively to the poorest of the poor that have been the responsibility of the hierarchical public bureaucracy and state owned public corporations. Therefore, the strength as argued in favour these third sector are social, political, economic and cultural point of view (ibid. 28-30; Chand 1999, 8; Panda 1987, 513-23; Nandedkar 1987, 468-72). The argument in favour of voluntary or non-governmental or third sector organisations for development has come in the forefront not only due to the failure of state or governmental machinery in the delivery of goods and services to the needy people but also due to the dramatic expansion of public responsibilities on the government – creation of the feeling of community belongingness – enabling civil organisations or NGOs in taking correct, timely and appropriate decisions in favour of local communities. Therefore as Kothari suggests that citizens groups have to be numerous and multifaceted to that the individual belongs not just one set of organisations ordained by the logic of the state or ruling party or opposition parties – but a whole spectrum of organisations (Kothari 1987, 438). Thus, the emergence or the development of the new partners in development which are nicknamed as social actors, development partners, alternatives, NGOs, voluntary organisations or in more sophisticated language - civil societies are a choice to the citizens for their association and involvement in a variety of ways.

POLITICAL TURN IN 1990 AND THE NGO SECTOR

The discussion in the above paragraphs clearly indicates that Nepal being a developing country could not remain isolated from global perspective of privatisation, market oriented economy, debureaucratisation and liberal democracy. As a result, after the readvent of democracy in 1990 and the formation of the government under the new constitutional framework of multiparty democracy, Nepali government also acted upon to pursue this new philosophy in development paradigm.

Soon after, Nepal again rehearsaled for the Eighth Plan (1992 – 97) where the government pronounced to a social and political process for mobilising and organising people relative to desired goals. This plan aimed at enhancing mass awareness and consciousness for self development and fostering civil responsibility and self reliance in conjunction with development initiatives at the community level (Eighth Plan Approach 1991, 9). Although the practice of social service and social development through non-governmental sector is age old in Nepal, it received new impetus only when country first experienced democratic practices in 1950-51. Till 1990, there were some few hundred NGOs registered under the Social Service Act. But after 1990 the government adopted a policy of minimum reliance on state control in economic affairs, disengagement and disinvestment from those fields where private sector can perform more efficiently without jeopardising social interest. For this the government shown commitment to create the necessary policy and implementation environment which would be conducive for the participation of the private sectors, the community and NGOs in development activities. The feeling behind this notion was that NGOs represent an important vehicle for carrying out development activities. Until 1990, peoples participation in development was an expression constantly used by political leaders and government functionaries to state propagated peoples participation. In fact, the Panchayat political thought was anchored on the peoples participation (Nepal South Asia Centre 1998, 138). Some programmes initiated during Panchayat like Small Farmers Development Programme (SFDP), Self-Reliance Development Programme (SDP), Community Forestry Projects (CFP) and Small Irrigation Projects (SIP) are noted for their achievement in social mobilisation (ibid.). However most of the participatory development programmes had disjointed endeavours into an institutional politico-development culture. The NGOs were embedded into quasi-governmental organisational frame work under the Social Service National Co-ordination Council headed by her Majesty the Queen. Absence of liberalisation in political expression led to state sponsored voluntarism where the concept of autonomy and institutionalisation of civil social structure remained mere mockery. As civil society aims at nurturing inspiration for social change in favour of human dignity and development. The realisation of this idea come into being only when democracy reinvented in Nepal.

PHENOMENAL GROWTH OF CIVIL SOCIETIES

Since 1990, the growth of civil association and NGOs sprung up as never before. These NGOs and social organisations grown in size and diversity covering various professions and occupations of trade unionism, human rights groups, taking special interest in the rights of women, children & disabled, corruption, environment conservation, etc. The following table is suffice to tell the strength of NGOs in Nepal.

| Sector | Region | | | | | |
	Far western	Mid Western	Western	Central	Eastern	Total
Child	2	3	6	363	16	390
Health	1	3	5	11	7	132
Disability	2	211	48	58	8	327
Com.Dev.	128	182	335	1398	291	2334
Women	12	32	112	293	55	504
Youth	27	50	169	591	101	938
Environment	3	20	35	200	26	284
Education	0	2	7	26	4	39
Aids	1	1	0	21	0	23
Moral Dev.	4	10	20	105	18	157
Total	180	514	737	3171	526	5128

Source: Nepal Human Development Report, 1998. P. 143.

The above table shows that the growth of NGOs in Nepal is phenomenal especially after the restoration of democracy in Nepal. Most of these are centred in Kathmandu and Pokhara and most of these are again centred with their activities in the sectors of women & child, community development, health & environment, etc. In the education sector only nominal number of NGOs are engaged. Interestingly the NGOs and civil organisations being engaged in policy advocacy and supportive to policy making are none. This seems that most of the NGOs or civil organisations are having their presence in the execution sector only.

DEVELOPMENT ISSUES AND SOCIAL STATUS IN NEPAL

Being mountainous and land-locked country Nepal is currently suffering from the problem of idea-lucked. Despite huge water resource, tourism, herbal & horticulture potentialities most the policy planners and policy executors are centred on to how to get maximum foreign aid and donations. As a result, vast resource potentiality of the country is still lying unused and unmobilised. The result is, out of total population 42% percent is below poverty line. Among them 17% are counted as the poorest. The population growth rate is 2.38% per annum. The contribution of agriculture in the total GDP remained 41.02% foreign assistance share is around 55% to the total development expenditure. The level of literacy is only 40%, only around 41% of rural population has access to primary health service. 4.9% of the total labour force is unemployed whereas 47 % is under employed. Around 80% of the total labour force is engaged in agriculture. Human resource is suffering from high birth rate, high child and mortality rate, low level of consumption and inappropriate mobilisation of human and natural resources. The enrolment in the primary, lower secondary and secondary level school is 69.4, 50.3 and 34.7%, respectively. Out of the total only 61% population have access to drinking water facilities and around 20% is served by sanitation facility. This scenario itself speaks the health of the capability of Nepali society to be able to be a good partner of socio-economic development with the government -- central and local.

WHY NEPAL FAILED IN PLANNED DEVELOPMENT ?

Till date, it was almost forgotten that the centre of development is the choice of people and their participation. Pursuit to national income was given top priority as it was an end itself. Also the failure of development, despite almost forty years of planned effort, is the result of (Dhakal 1997, 4-7; The Ninth Plan 1997-2002; 1998, 27-28):
- - lack of long term vision is development plan;
- - lack of human resource planning;
- - lack of co-ordination in using foreign aid and inabilities to fix

- priorities while drawing such aid;
- lack of strong legal background in supporting development ;
- lack of effective monitoring and evaluation system in plan implementation;
- lack of relationship between research and training and national priorities;
- lack of accountability and transparency in transaction of development works;
- lack of people's mobilisation of self-help basis, under utilisation of
- resources and tendency of over-dependence on the government.

The developmental effort, thus made during the forty years, was suffered immensely due to the various reasons. People's participation was limited to labour participation. The organic growth and development of the people's organisations were often disallowed due to one party dominated closed political system. The absence of liberalism in political domain affected regularly to the rightful mobilisation of social organisations and their institutionalisation. Pseudo democratic behaviour of the rulers made mockery to the transparency and accountability. This culture is still dominant in the administrative arena of Nepal.

NEPALESE THRUST OF DEVELOPMENT FOR THE COMING DAYS

Poverty alleviation and raising the level of the standard of people is being major goal of development plan of Nepal, the government has identified some strategies in this direction. Such strategies are (see e.g. Ninth Plan 1998, 72-73):
- Integrated development of agriculture and forestry,
- Industrial development on the basis of competitive advantages,
- Reduction of social and economic inequalities through social and economic development,
- Enhancement of co-operatives as a means of development,
- Liberal and market oriented economic system
- Enable institutions to take leadership in development,
- Decentralisation and democratisation,
- Development of human resources for high and sustainable growth, and
- Expansion of education and family planning activities so as to build up.awareness of the society

Thus, the planning goal of Ninth Plan is to be achieved through the development and expansion of social capital, which, as the Plan stressed, would help to enabling social institutions and enhance autonomy. Economic reform, competitive market, development of social services targeting poor and downtrodden, decentralised decision marketing process with the involvement of more and more people at grass-root level, and giving more autonomy are some of the strategic targets set by the government so that it can create an autonomous civil society. The government thus, intends to utilise comparative ability of Non governmental organisations using a process of peoples empowerment.

However, the question of transparency in transaction of their business and accountability towards tax payers is being increasingly felt for the operation of NGOs. (see Dhakal 1999, NPC 1998, 753-54). Time and again various issue are realised against NGOs (Dhakal 1988, 27-35) and their sincerity in development efforts from the government side. NGOs are regarded as vehicles of development and pins high hopes on their strengths and efficiency (Rising Nepal 1997, Dec. 29). Even some acclaimed INGOs advocated NGOs have really woke up the society from its slumber of ignorance and have injected in it the much needed enthusiasm and encouragement. Despite haring so much about the success of NGOs, why is the country still mired in poverty and backwardness? Are they not the additional cause to further the gap between rich and poor? These are the questions that need to be timely addressed, if NGOs well driven to materialise the idea that development causes through peoples participation.

THE ISSUES RAISED AGAINST NGOS

Academicians and professionals engaged in the area of NGOs are quite aware that the organisation of plural society or NGOs are not free from pejorative. These are:

- NGOs are organised for the furtherance of personal aid family interest and lack dedicated personalities,
- NGOs are parasites, capable of surviving only on aid money,
- They are gobbling foreign money there by helping inflation rate which has already hit the economy,
- most of the fund allocated to NGOs goes to administrative and other procedural expenses unaccountable neither toward public, nor to the government. Their financial activities are not transparent,
- They have no grass-root base and are run from distant urban posh areas (Post and Preuss 1998, 4) out of the purview of work evaluation.

If the government, as stated in the policy predicaments for the development of Nepal, and the society is going to be highly depended on NGOs as real partners some of the aforementioned issues have to be addressed in time.

THE INITIATION PROCESS OF EMPOWERMENT

The government is trying to make these civil organisations as transparent, accountable and efficient in resource mobilisation. The first step taken so far is that before renewal of NGO from district office, it has to submit auditing report and the source of fund they use. This will help NGOs accountable and transparent in their activities. Even the local self government act 1998 makes it mandatory to the local government authorities (VDCs, DDCs and Municipalities) to work in close co-operation with NGOs and consumer societies (see Local Self Government Act 1998, 98-100). The Act say that local government and NGOs or consumer societies at respected areas will minimise duplication of work, funding and will maintain a close co-ordination while working for local development. The co-operation will be taken in planning implementation and management and assessment and evaluation of the projects launched in the local level. However, the accounting and recording of the expenses has made mandatory. Also local government will encourage NGOs in identification of the problem, planning, implementation, evaluation and monitoring of any of the local projects. Even the Ninth Plan purports to encourage NGOs to be able to efficiently allocating the resources of the local bodies which are considered as people's representative organisations (Ninth Plan 1998, 747).

The users group as stated in the Ninth Plan, will be capacitated with training on how to use authority and duties similarly. These organisations will also be trained to maintain projects. Thus the NGOs or civil organisations in any form are made active partners of local authorities and development.

In the process of capacity building and empowerment to make these civil organisations autonomous and active, many international donor agencies involvement is noticeable. DANIDA, USAID, GTZ are some of them. DANIDA, a new entrant in co-operation is involved in electoral reforms, local self government and training of public officials on democracy and human rights. GTZ is engaged primarily in urban development, community participation, environment management, small scale industries and self-help organisations. However, the assistance is available only on the fulfilment of these conditions:

- rule of law;
- human rights;
- political participation;
- open market system; and
- development oriented state actions.

While USAID has focused on sustained economic development, increasing of democratic participation, protection of human rights, legitimate government behaviour and the augmentation of fundamental human rights. Thus, in the process of institutionalisation and empowerment of the civil society, all NGOs and INGOs are mobilised and directed to modernise state institutions, create force to capable and active for economic reforms and redefine state society relationship for good governance (Dahal 1996, 8).

Special programmes have been envisaged to make better and more participation of women and backward ethnic groups in decision process by providing them appropriate training programmes and representing them in various local agencies, making personnel service (local) responsible towards public, and establishing an effective monitoring and evaluation system representing civil societies. This will ensure the empowerment of the civil society towards building an autonomous society.

CONCLUSION

Development is possible only with the co-operative efforts of the government, private and non-governmental sector. In order to speed up economic and social development activities of the country, non governmental sector have already been involved as the strong and effective partner. Nepal's development issue that brew up from poverty, and low social capacity can be addressed only when the civil societies are well capacitated, co-ordinated, transparent and accountable. Area specialisation, maintaining efficiency at all levels, identification and mobilisation of resources at the maximum possible extent, simplicity in administration, perfect monitoring and evaluation system has to be observed in the running and functioning if the civil societies are to be an equal partner of development. Competitiveness is a must to address social and economical issues.

The policy documents of the government are fully oriented to empower civil societies and necessary steps for legal reforms have been carried on so as to make these civil societies' development practices. The mushroom growth of NGOs in Nepal speaks only about the quantitative growth, but does not ensure their capacity to furthering the development thrust of Nepal. Also the patronisation and grabbing resources without social accountability may lead to widen the gap of 'have' and 'have-nots' in coming days. Therefore, a harmonious balance between NGOs, government and private organisations becomes necessary. Democracy, decentralisation and autonomous civil society can be materialised only when society through social organisations becomes competent.

REFERENCES

Adhikari, Ambika Prasad (1998): *Urban and Environmental Planning in Nepal.* Kathmandu: IUCN

Chand, Diwakar (1998): The Role of Civil Society in Democratisation: NGO Perspective. In Shrestha, Ananda (ed.): *The Role of Civil Society and Democratisation in Nepal.* Kathmandu: NEFAS, FES

Aditya, Anand (ed.): *The Role of Civil Society and Democratisation in Nepal.* Kathmandu: NEFAS, FES

Chand, Diwakar (1999): '*Non-Governmental Organisations in Development*', a seminar paper presented in a Seminar organised by Central Department of Public Administration, T.U., Kathmandu

Chitrakar, Anil (1996): *Working with NGOs.* Kathmandu: IUCN

Dahal, Devraj (1996): *The Challenges of Good Governance: Decentralisation and*

Development in Nepal, Kathmandu: Centre for Governance and Development Studies

Dhakal, Govind Pd (1988): Role of Voluntary Organisations in Urban Development. *Prashasan.* 53rd Issue, November

Dhakal, Tek Nath (1999): Dynamics and Drawbacks of SWCs Promotional Support to NGOs in Nepal. *PAAN* Vol. 8 & 9, Year 5, January/February/June/July

Elsenhans, Hartmut (1997): *"Politico-economic Foundation of the Empowerment of the Citizens and an Autonomous Civil Society".* Seminar Paper Presented in the XVIIth World Congress IPSA RC4, Seoul, Korea 17 - 21August

HMG/N – NPC. 1998. *The Ninth Plan (1997-2002).* Kathmandu: NPC.

HMG/N Ministry of Law and Justice. *"Local Self Government Act 1998"* in *Collection of Acts 1999 Part I,* Kathmandu: HMG/N Ministry of Law and Justice, Law Book Management Committee.

HMG/N, NPC. 1989. *Programme for the Fulfilment of Basic Needs (1985 – 2000).* Kathmandu: NPC.

HMG/N, NPC. 1991. *Approach to the Eighth Plan 1992-1997.* Kathmandu: His Majesty's Government, NPC.

Hossain, Farhad and Myllylä, Susanna (1998): Non-Governmental Organisations: In Search of Theory and Practice. In Hossain, F. & Myllylä, S. (eds.): *NGOs Under Challenge: Dynamics and Drawbacks in development.* Helsinki: Ministry for Foreign Affairs of Finland, Department of International Development Cooperation

Kothari, Rajani (1987): Voluntary Organisations in a Plural Society. *Indian Journal of Public Administration,* Vol. XXXIII, No. 3, July-September

Lee, Han Been (1959): *Future Innovation and Development,* Seoul: Panmun

Mälkiä, Matti & Hossain, Farhad (1998): Changing Patterns of Development Co-operation Conceptualising Non-Governmental Organisations in Development. In Hossain, F. & Myllylä, S. (eds.): *NGOs Under Challenge: Dynamics and Drawbacks in development.* Helsinki: Ministry for Foreign Affairs of Finland, Department of International Development Cooperation

Nandedkar, V. G. (1987): Voluntary Associations: A Strategy in Development. *Indian Journal of Public Administration,* Vol. XXXIII, No. 3, July-September

Nepal South Asia Centre (1998): *Nepal Human Development Report 1998.* Prepared under the aegis of UNDP. Kathmandu: UNDP

Panda, Snehalata (1987): Social Transformation and Voluntary Agencies: A Model. *Indian Journal of Public Administration,* Vol. XXXIII, No. 3, July-September

Post, Uli & Hans-Joachim, Preuss (1998): The Challenges Facing NGOs. *The Rising Nepal,* Feb. 14

Robinson, Mark (1996): Governance. In: Kuper, Adam & Kuper, Jessica (eds.): *The Social Science Encyclopedia*, London: Routledge

11. NEPALI NGOS COMBATING TRAFFICKING OF GIRLS AND WOMEN

Shanti Bajracharya Rajbhandari

INTRODUCTION

The status of women is exceptionally low in Nepal by any international standard. Nepal is one of the few countries in the world where the life expectancy for women is lower than that for men. Female life expectancy is 53.7 years where as male life expectancy is 55.2 years. Female literacy rate is 25 per cent.

Trafficking of girls and women to India for sex work is a serious problem relating to the low status of women in Nepali society. Women and girls are trafficked out of the country forcibly or by giving them false promises. It is estimated that every year 5.000-7.000 girls from Nepal enter illegally the sex trade in India and that at least 100,000 Nepali women work in Indian brothels. A number of Nepali girls are also trafficked to Saudi Arabia. The trafficked girls generally belong to the hill communities like Tamang, Magar, Gurung, Damai, Kami besides some from the supposed privileged communities like Brahmin and Chetris and others.

Government and NGOs have undertaken different preventive and controlling activities to stop the trade and to eradicate it from the society. For example, in the criminal code there is a provision for punishment of up to 20 years imprisonment for traffickers. However, there is lack of law enforcement and lack of co-ordination and co-operation among NGOs. Although trafficking is a national problem deserving high priority, none of the governments formed after the restoration of democracy in 1990 have given the issue due priority.

Many NGOs have been active on the issue of trafficking and turned it into a major issue during the past decade. Though the voice against trafficking has reached grass root level it has not been abble to reduced it. Reduction in the registration of cases against trafficking is not a proof of reduction in trafficking.

In this paper facts are presented on the basis of observation of three NGOs, namely ABC Nepal, Maiti Nepal and CWIN. Their head offices and field offices have been visited, conversation with chairman, Durga Ghimire, ABC Nepal, Anuradha Koirala, Chairman Maiti Nepal, Mr, Gauri Pradhan chairman CWIN as well as members and volunteers of the NGOs have been conducted. Moreover, local news papers, published books and booklets have been reviewed. It was not possible to interview on real victims but Rehabilitation centres at Kakervitta and Rani Biratnager were briefly observed.

TRAFFICKING SITUATION IN NEPAL

People generally confuse trafficking with prostitution. These two words are related only to the extent that women and girls are trafficked to be sold for the purpose of prostitution. But one should not forget that trafficking is forcibly and unlawfully trapping women and girls, who are then sold in the market whereas prostitution may be compelled, under duress or even voluntary and for different personal reasons including financial. It is true that trafficking occurs all over the world in different forms and the concept of trafficking differs in different countries. In some cases men, women and children are trafficked for exchange and selling of body parts, in some places for the illegal adoption, repayment of debt and mostly to be sold in the sex market for forced prostitution.

In the case of Nepal, women and girls are trafficked for prostitution in different Indian brothels and abroad. Those who are trafficked are either forcibly taken or trapped or lured with false promises. Trafficking of women and girls for prostitution is internationally recognised as a violent and cruel form of crime. Trafficking should be defined in the national context. It should be separated from prostitution as prostitution is only one of the many factors that initiates trafficking. Prostitution is as a form of work that may be based on the individual's own choice whereas trafficking of girls and women is seen as a more violent and enforced prostitution.

This trade is expanding due to commercialisation and threatens to change it into industry. Some of the people engage in trafficking and prostitution business claim that it is their right to have legal license for their living. Globalisation and liberalisation of markets also forces people to earn in one's own manner where there is lack of resources. That must be challenged for NGOs to work against trafficking. At times, an argument is put forward, that everybody has a right to earn in one's own way. So the prostitution and trafficking is part of it. But the commercialisation of trafficking breaks down social values, dignity and human rights of girls, women and children. So the argument should not be in favour of trafficking for prostitution and licensing system.

The problem of trafficking in girls is on the rise in the districts adjoining Kathmandu. Particularly, girls and women in the age group 12 to 32 years are at risk of being sold. Now this problem is affecting nearly all the districts of Nepal. Efforts on the part of NGOs as well as the government at saving the women from this danger is highly needed. NGOs, by their nature, can be effective in this regard. However, the problem itself is highly complicated. Trafficking in women now seems to have taken a shape of commercial enterprise, making it all the more serious. Some women NGOs have as initial steps against the problems, taken rigorous campaign on the issue. However, there is no reliable figure from the government or other official sources as to the exact number of women that have been sold. Therefore, it is necessary to rely on the figures provided by studies of the social workers who are actively engaged in movement against such trafficking.

The situation analysis on children and women of Nepal, prepared jointly by the National Planning Commission/HMG and the UNICEF in 1992 has mentioned trafficking and prostitution as a big problem. The report also makes a note of the failure in implementation of legal provisions to help girls and women at such risks besides commending the acitive role of NGOs in this issue. Girl trafficking and prostitution is another hidden problem in the growing number of Nepalese girls and women who end up in the brothels on Indian cities, especially Bombay. Trafficking in women and children both internally and across Indo-Nepal border for commercial sexual exploitation has become a serious issue in the Nepalese society these days.

The Women Development Division of the Ministry of Labour and Social Welfare has been running a skill development programme for the victims of the problem areas. But of course, such a programme, however welcome and needed, is insignificant in comparison to the needs.

It is becoming to the surface as Nepali girls and women are returning home from the brothels of India or being returned to Nepal because of HIV infection.

Thus, various NGOs working on women and girls trafficking are trying to become better informed and take serious actions against this problem. It is estimated that at least 8-10% of Nepal's population must know about and tens of thousands are actively involved in this illegal, and in terms of forced prostitution, in human behaviour.

The districts of Nepal that are most inflicted with the problem of girls trafficking with a vast majority of reported cases occuring are Makwanpur, Nuwakot, Dhading, Sindhupalchok, Kavre, Rupendehi, Kaski, Sunsari, Rosuwa, Nawalparasi, Udaypur and Jhapa. In 1994, with the help of UNICEF a joint awareness campaign was launched by the Nepal Police, the students of Padmakanye Campus in Kathmandu and Maiti Nepal against girl trafficking in villages most severely aflicted with the problem. The response was said to be very encouraging.

CAUSES CONTRIBUTING TO TRAFFICKING IN GIRLS AND WOMEN AND THEIR SALE IN SEX MARKET

A multiple factors seem to be at play in contributing to the origin and sustenance of the problem of the girl trafficking, of course poverty and its consequence, unwanted migration in search for work and livelihood is an underlying one that makes women most vulnerable to the lure from unscrupulous elements. Besides, there is also a reduced access for girls to education and other opportunities. The following as the main factors behind the trafficking of women from Nepal to brothels in India and Arabian countries: absolute poverty, low status of girl child, lack of employment opportunities, tradition and culture, impact of modernisation, open border, lack of political commitment, lack of implementation of anti-trafficking laws and a highly lucrative business.

However, the reasons for the situation are not limited to factors mentioned above. All the girls sold into the trade are not tricked. Many are knowingly and in concurrence with the family and the community forced into the situation so that they can help improve family's financial condition. This has further complicated the problem. And even the NGOs have not extended their efforts to try to solve this aspect of trafficking. Also, women who have returned from brothels wish to continue and extend the trade, encourage girls and women in their family and the neighbourhood to join the profession by offering the poverty stricken women to have a good life. This has contributed to the increase in the number of source districts despite NGOs efforts at discouraging trafficking.

The open border with India is a major hindrance at eradicating such trafficking, the demand for Nepalese girls in the neighbouring countries seem to be on the rise. Open border makes it impossible for the resource-constrained agencies to try and to stop of the unwanted flow.

Political, social, religious, cultural factors and the involvement of organised crime are also responsible besides economic conditions. The growing influence of the internet and the pornographic films and publications is extending the trafficking business. Society's traditional concept of "owning" their women is at the root of the problem of sale and trafficking in women.

We are also facing very strong invisible market forces (strong demand and strong supply) that drive the whole trafficking process. The whole situation looks like a stand still now, not knowing what to do or where to start, because the ruler community is also helpless, the victims are totally lost and confused about what they are in, while those law enforcement authorities are not well aware, equipped, or enforced to take the necessary preventive and enforcement measures. This is not only a national problem, trafficking of women and children out of Nepal to other destinations has become an international issue.

It is estimated that 66.% of the commercial sex workers were involved in this trade out of their own wish, 38 % influenced by female friends, and 9 % influenced by natal family members, 6. % by pimps, 4 % by brothel owners, 4. % influenced by mothers, and 2 % were found to be involved in it because they were Deukies and Badis.

NGOs EFFORTS

Against above mentioned background many NGOs are working to solve the problem of girls trafficking. The task, however difficult it may be has attracted untiring attention in quite of few NGOs which are seriously working on it.

NGOs are turning trafficking from a non-issue to a major issue. Though the voice against trafficking has reached the grassroot level the NGOs haven't been able to reduce the problem. Nepali NGOs have been continuously fighting against this problem for the past ten years. NGOs have done a lot to minimise this problem with efforts such as rehabilitation of the victims and nation-wide awareness programme. They have also taken up programmes for making women economically independent, training for women, special education for the girls child and the establishment of prevention homes.

Some NGOs have undertaken different preventive and controlling methods involving rescue operations, rehabilitation, awareness and sensitisation programmes in the risk areas to negate entry of new entrants. NGOs' pressure group has also formulated networking groups to pressure the government and develop an intelligence network with efficient networking collaboration among countries of the region.

One of the most successful intervention programmes by NGOs was the repatriation of 120 minor girls from Bombay in July 1996. That year on Februaty 5, the police in the Indian state of Maharastra raided several brothels in Bombay and saved 487 minor girls of which 228 were of Nepali origin. The Government of Maharastra brought all the saved girls before the Juvenile Justice Board and redeemed them into various observation homes in Bombay. Then they approached government of Nepal for the girls repatriation. When there was no response and immediate action on the part of the Nepalese Government, the Maharastra authorities as well as some local NGOs working for the prevention and rehabilitation of the minor girls approached Nepali NGOs. Various NGOs working for the prevention of girls trafficking and the children's rights immediately made the Prime Minister of Nepal to demand immediate action on the plight of Nepalese girls in Maharastra. The Nepalese NGO activists also met various other ministers on the subject only to be disappointed. Finally, with no active help from the government the NGOs collaborated to have the girls stranded in Maharastra, then repatriated home safely in Nepal and rehabilitated. For this purpose, a team of social workers visited Maharastra at the invitation of the Department of Women and Children of the Government of Maharastra. There were 228 registered girls in February 12, 1996. They were housed at different centres on May 20, 1996 when the Nepalese social workers got there only 201 remained there, 3 had died of medical reasons and some had run away while a number of them had been handed over to the guardians. The Nepalese team brought 120 remaining girls back to Nepal and housed them at various facilities in Kathmandu such as indicated in the Table 1.

Table 1: Sheltering of returned sex workers from Bombay in 1996

Name of the NGO	Number of people
Maiti Nepal	30
ABC Nepal	27
CWIN	24
WOREC	14
Nawajyoti	14
Shanti Punarsthapana	13
Stri Shakti	8

Source: Gauri Pradha: Back Home From Brothels

MAJOR NGOS ON THE SCENE

There are more than hundred NGOs working against the exploitation of women and children. Each and every NGO's success depends upon its purpose and the kind of people running it. ABC Nepal and Maiti Nepal are two well known and successful NGOs working on women's issues and girls' trafficking. Even these NGOs are subjected to criticism.

ABC Nepal

ABC Nepal is shortened form for Agroforestry, Basic Health and Cooperatives. It a leading NGO working for uplifting girls and women in Nepal. It was established in 1987. It has been working to spread awareness, sensitising women, and stopping girls' trafficking before 1990. In the beginning it was established with the objective of promoting agroforestry, basic health facilities and to form women's cooperative by involving the local women in income generating programme. Gradually this NGO gather village experiences and realised that girls and women are in serious trouble. They were trafficked and sold in brothels in India at different prices like commodities. The cause was primarily poor economy of the villagers, ignorance and illiteracy among village women. Then this NGO changed its objective a little to concentrate on girls' trafficking, prostitution and AIDS. It started to put pressure on the government and the public for controlling illegal flesh trade and trafficking.

In 1990 ABC Nepal conducted a national workshop to create wide spread awareness on the issue. Probably it was the first important open discussion on trafficking issue. The traffickers are believed to be protected by politicians. Organising such an open workshop needs a great courage. ABC Nepal jointly with Women Awareness Centre (WAC) Nepal organised a two-day seminar titled 'Towards Equal Power: South Asian Women's Voice' in August 1995 aiming at highlighting the need to political empowerment of women. The seminar formed an eleven-member national pressure group and village level pressure groups in nine villages.

ABC Nepal has also produced various materials and street drama to make people more aware about the problem. Some of the activities and materials produced by it are

1. Booklets on girls trafficking and AIDS.
2. The study report of girls trafficking in Ichowk and Mahankal villages of Nepal.
3. Two different kinds of audio cassettes on girls trafficking.
4. Skill development training programme, specially sewing classes and also sponsored literacy classes.
5. Rehabilitation centre to house rescued girls.
6. Formation of women's saving and credit programme groups and launching of health camps.

ABC Nepal has been launching its programmes in Kathmandu, Nuwakot, Nawalparasi, Ramechap, Dhading and Sindhupalchowk districts and Bhatrabas and Danchi VDCs. These are adjoining districts and villages of Kathmandu, the capital district and are affected by girls trafficking problem.

ABC is very active in raising women's voice and issues by launching work shops, national and village level seminars, participating in international seminars, forming different pressure groups and keeping documents. To control and prevent girls and women trafficking Mrs. Durga Ghimire the Chairperson of ABC Nepal expresses the need for national commitment and social awareness among all Nepalese people.

The success of this NGO can be credited to its systematic management with seven-member management body. Mrs. Ghimire and Ms Meera Arjyal are the founders. This executive body provides policy guidelines. It also has 2600 women volunteers all over its project areas. There are fifteen full time staff at ABC Nepal central office in Kathmandu. Its major donors are currently CEDPA (Centre for Development and Population Activities), Plan International and UNESCO/Japan.

Some villagers criticise ABC Nepal calling it *banar NGO,* noise making NGO and money making NGO. To judge a NGO one needs to study it in depth but ABC's critics seem to criticising mainly because most villagers do not like talking about women's issues in their village. Also NGO working on girls' and women's trafficking, violence against women, women's empowerment comes as a challenge for traffickers. However, this NGO is actively working on women's issues and development since before the restoration of democracy in Nepal in 1990. It seems a little bit stagnant at the grassroot level, especially in the case of girls' trafficking. But ABC managed to document and publish education materials on HIV/AIDS and girls' trafficking and issues related to women. The most important work ABC has undertaken, however, seems to be forming and coordinating of network groups against girls' trafficking.

Maiti Nepal

Literary meaning of Maiti Nepal in Nepali is parental home of any married women or mother's home where a married woman can have shelter when she is in trouble. Maiti Nepal is purely women's NGO established in April 1993 with the initiative of Ms. Anuradha Koirala. It has made its mark in the society in a very short time. In recognition to her work Ms. Corolla won the social welfare award of the year 1998 from Social Welfare Council, Nepal. She comes with experience from social work and NGO's oppression from ABC Nepal.

Maiti Nepal started with small groups of street girls and a seed money of Rs 900 each for Nanglo shops. Nanglo shop is a traditional low-end street shop selling tobacco and tid bits. The organisation started to rehabilitate street girls providing them with safe home. Maiti Nepal works at the grassroots level with deprived, victimised, exploited and the girls and women rescued from trafficking and/or returning from brothels in India. The other objective of it is to check, control and take action against the traffickers who sell these women with false promises of marriage, luring them or fake job with attractive salary and travelling opportunities in foreign countries. Besides, Maiti Nepal provides shelter for single women parents in critical circumstances. It also provides hostel facilities for HIV/AIDS infected people who are rejected by the society. No number of HIV/AIDS patients is rising so Maiti Nepal decided to try to solve the problem at the source.

In 1994 Maiti Nepal started a campaign against women's and girl's trafficking in Nuwakot, Sindhupalchowk, Makwanpur, Rasuwa, Dhading, Newalparasi, Udaypur, Jhapa, Itahari, Dharan and Kakarvitta. This campaign was actively supported and participated in by UNICEF, Nepal Police, and the teachers and students of Padmakanya Campus, girls' college in Kathmandu.

According to the director of Maiti Nepal, Ms. Anuradha Koirala, social work has no limits so she will accept to help needy people even if they are out of their objective and the target group. Moreover, they have to face challenge as people instead of willing to accept the magnitude of the problem engaged in a lot of controversy. But the trafficking trade is rapidly growing in Nepal. It has reached a level beyond repairs and if action is not taken in time, it might be an irreparable loss. Recently Maiti Nepal has started a programme called Students Against Girls Trafficking in the most affected districts of Sindhupalchowk and Nuwakot.

Maiti Nepal has enjoyed international limelight. It was a moment of special pleasure and pride for Maiti Nepal that Prince Charles of United Kingdom visited the organisation in February 1998 and met with HIV/AIDS patients. The Prince announced help to Maiti Nepal offering proceeds from the sales of 500 of his own paintings. The amount collected from the sale of the paintings was 67 275 pounds was handed over to the Chairperson and Director Ms. Anurahda Koirala by Mr. Peter Higgins, the Deputy Head of Mission at the British Embassy in Nepal in September 1998.

Maiti Nepal first gained international exposure when The Washington Post published a news about the visit to Maiti Nepal by the First Lady Hillary Clinton of United States in 1995 and provided some financial support to develop and expand its activities. The funds thus received will be invested in strengthening Maiti Nepal with its own hostel buildings. It has also a plan to build a hospital and a rehabilitation centre for HIV/AIDS victims, Hepatitis B and Tuberculosis, and a plan to add a transit home in Biratnagar and a rehabilitation centre in Ithaca. It also has a plan to educate the girls at border points to create more awareness about trafficking.

Radd Barn, a Norwegian NGO, also financed the centre. ILO pays the salaries for the working staff. Another INGO CARNG helps them to sponsor street girls, child workers in the carpet and the garment factories as well as do some individual sponsors.

Maiti Nepal perfumes its functions based on participatory approach, hearing and sharing from grassroot level and volunteers. It follows button up approach. It has a informal body consisting of follow Chairman and Director, Vice Chairman, Lawyer, Account and Shelter In-charge. There are also some volunteers

Maiti Nepal has three Transit Homes in the border areas of Kakervitta, Birganj and Sunauli to prevent girls and track the traffickers. These transit homes provide short period safe transit shelter home for victims. The number of victims of HIV/AIDS, other diseases, rescued girls and deprived women, girls and children are increasing in Maiti Nepal. In 1999 there were 370 victims permanently living with Maiti Nepal. As the number of victim is increasing the burden is also getting on Maiti Nepal. So, Maiti Nepal made opened its doors for any body willing to participate in income generating and non formal education programmes of Maiti Nepal. It also lunched a micro credit programme for girls and provided loan for 25 small street shops for destitute women. Maiti Nepal is supporting 150 girls by providing education sponsorship programme. It has also established a pre-primary school named Teresa Academy for children residing at it's Kathmandu rehabilitation center. Thus Maiti Nepal is working very hard to uplift deprived girls, women and children. Maiti Nepal is in the fore front of anti-trafficking activities and is acclaimed nationally and internationally. But for this organisation to maintain its stature it still needs to observe some of fundamental principles of NGOs such as transparency, accountability and self evaluation.

CHALLENGES FOR THE CONCERNED NGOS

NGOs, whether good or bad have not escaped criticism. NGOs have to take these criticisms in a positive way. It is a medium from which they learn the ways of being sustainable NGOs. The common challenges facing ABC /NEPAL and Maiti Nepal can be seen from two sides, within the NGO and out side the NGO.

Challenges within organisation:

- Problems in operation: NGOs management have many problems. NGOs seen to be confused as to where it is better to run under a charismatic personality or an organised body of individuals. Among the two NGOs mentioned here, ABC Nepal seem to be doing all right as an organised body of individuals while Maiti Nepal is run under the charismatic stewardship of Ms. Anuradha Koirala.

- Problems in policy formation: The confusion as stated above seem to have direct bearing on policy formulation of on NGO. The NGOs operating as a body of individuals seem to be some what systematic in their policy in comparison to the individual-led NGO which betrays a tendency for fluctuation in policy. This shows problems of continuity in NGOs.

- Transparency: Like often sectors in Nepalese officialdom, these NGOs also do not seem to be free from "the lack of transparency", when the project is run with the funds from local sources, these NGOs like others, seem to be simple and transparent. They tend to be less so when they start to run with foreign contribution. Many a clashes within the NGOs that have occurred seem to have origin in this fact. And this gives rise to a glaring example of a problem of sustainability.

- Size and capacity: The challenges facing the NGOs is also closely linked with their size and capacity. Because they are easy and uncomplicated to work with people prefer to come to them to have their problems redressed. The people seeking help do not know about the size and capacity of the NGO. Ms. Anuradha Koirala's experience is very telling in this regard when they at Maiti Nepal realized that it was not enough just providing shelter to girls because people started bringing in lost children found wondering aimlessly in the streets of Nepal.

- Struggle for funding: NGOs are formed with some objectives in mind. They have the knowledge about local needs. At times, when they are struggling to find funds, they have to compromise with the interest of a donor who may be willing to support but has a different objective. Many a times there is a rise of a local NGO drifting completely from its original objectives.

- Volunteerism: Unlike governments, NGOs' work is mostly need-based and thus effective as it satisfies immediate need. The workers here also have to work efficiently and on their toes. But how long can one work as a volunteer at nominal pay. To expect efficiency and effectiveness on a long term basis from a volunteer is impractical. For this reason, also modern NGOs, at least some of them, have developed into professional organisation and voluntarism is becoming a bigger challenge. Maiti Nepal and ABC Nepal are experiencing a need for some kind of pay for people working there although they expect to continue to attract volunteers to work for short periods and just for pocket money.

Challenges from outside:

- Political patronage: Often NGO initiatives result in arrest of people involved in flesh trade and trafficking. But most of them are set free even before the legal proceedings have begun, chiefly on account of political interference and pressures. In such a condition, NGOs find working very difficult. For example arrested brothel owners running flesh trade involving minor girls have been released under heavy political pressure after one week of his arrest.

- Media creates negative impact on society: At times, media, instead of covering NGO activities publicises victims. This has shown to result in the victim getting mistreatment in society forcing them to return to the work they so desperately seek to leave behind. NGOs also feel bad as they do not receive the credit for good work that they deserve.

- Lucrative business: Stopping trafficking and rehabilitating the girls rescued is getting more and more complicated because high profitability of the operation (Rs 20 000 to Rs 40 000 of easy money) has made the operators run their business more professionally. People tend to think of it less as a crime and more as a business. This is making it spreading instead of declining it.

- Lack of firm government policy: The constitution of Nepal 1990 prohibited the trafficking of human beings. New civil code made in 1987, traffickers can be sentenced in 20 years of imprisonment. Despite these provisions, the implementation of law is not effective and has no significant change in the life of destitute girls and women. The government officials and the police admit that there is a practical difficulty in arresting and charging an individual before the actual crime, only on suspicion.

- Bilateral cooperation needed: The open border between India and Nepal has made women trafficking easy. Therefore, there should be bilateral talk between India and Nepal for this trafficking to stop.

- Money defining social standing: In many districts, going abroad to make money has become a matter of prestige and pride. In the villages of Ichowk, Duachaur, Haibung and Tarke Ghang etc. in Sindhupalchowk district, girls themselves initiate the process of this trade with their full knowledge. NGOs have paid a lot of attention in this areas but still people there take going abroad in this connection no less dignified.

- Parental attention: Many parents in villages infected with this problem hand over their daughters to the brokers and agents in the hope that their daughters will return as rich women. Efforts of NGOs alone in stopping, where parent's themselves are active participants in the trade, are almost impossible.

- Society's perception of NGOs: The popular perception prevailing in society that NGOs are active in this field basically to attract foreign money has done little to put the issues at centre stage. Even responsible government, ministers and officials are found insensitively making remarks about NGOs being over smart and trying to be parallel to government and making Nepal a dumping site for AIDS etc.

- Little concern among those who can make a change:

    The society, including the members who can make a change like the police, judges and politicians have taken the problem as a fact of life with little thought on how they can contribute in eradicating this evil. This apathy on the of society the must glaring in the spreading of the problem.

SUGGESTIONS

1. The NGOs currently working on the issues of girls trafficking seem to be concentrating on the case of girls and women tricked into the situation. This is only one aspect of the problem as the larger picture involves girls and women sold or forced into the sex market knowingly and with consent either by themselves or their family especially because of the poverty and/or inability to repay dept. Therefore, NGOs in their attempt at anti-trafficking measures first need to extend the definition of trafficking itself.

2. Reliability of various studies can be questioned as data presented by different organisation on the issue seem to vary significantly. Therefore, there is a need to base arguments on the basis of in depth field study.

3. NGOs should aim at investing the funds received from donors in appropriate ventures so that most can be made from such funds.

4. NGOs at times seem to make unrealistic promises. They should promise to deliver only to the extent of their capability and try to deliver it. In absence of such the society will place the blame on NGOs themselves and the problem will stay as it is.

5. There is a great need to involve local agencies and people in NGO efforts at forming pressure groups and implementing anti-trafficking programmes.

6. The problem of trafficking is there mainly because of poverty, lack of education, ignorance and unemployment in rural areas. Without targeting these causes the problem is unlikely to be addressed effectively. The NGOs therefore need to invest in creating employment opportunities in the risk areas in addition to spreading their information and awareness campaigns in such problematic and infested areas.

7. As the problem of trafficking is not confined to national boundaries the government and non-government agencies should conduct trafficking control and prevention programmes jointly with governments and NGO in the neighbouring countries.
8. The NGOs need to join hands in opposing and eliminating political patronage to people profiting from this unlawful trade besides campaigning further stringent laws and implementing them.
9. As a large number of returnees are believed to lure innocent girls into the market, such returnees should be helped to reunite with their families or rehabilitate into the society so that they have less incentive to carry on the trade they have left behind.

CONCLUSION

No doubt the voice and efforts of NGOs are very important in eradicating trafficking of girls and women. But at the same time, NGOs are also facing different challenges. Instead of decline and control of girls and women trafficking in most affected districts the menace is spreading to additional number of districts. It is not possible to control this rising trend just by the NGOs mainly because the problem encompasses a wide range of socio-cultural, educational, economic and international factors. Co-operation and effective involvement of government, NGOs, society, donors and other international agencies can only make real difference in the problem of trafficking. Each of them need to get involved keeping in mind their own strengths and weaknesses.

REFEFENCES

ABC Nepal Annual Report 1996-1997 (1997) Kathmandu: ABC Nepal..

Acharya, Meena (1994) *The statistical profile of Nepalese Women.* Kathmandu: I IDS

Adhikari, Radha (1997) *Nepal's lost daughters, India's soiled goods: An analysis of returned sex worker's situation in Nepal.* MSc Health Promotions Sciences (Policy Report). London: London School of Hygiene and Tropical Medicine.

Bhattachan K.B and Mishara Chaitnya (1997) *Development practices in Nepal.* Kathmandu: FES.

Marilyan Carr, Martha Chen, Rena Thabvala (1997) *Speaking out women's Economic empowerment in South Asia.*

Pradhan G .- *Nepalma Chelibetiko Deha Byapar Yathartha tatha Chunautiharu-B.S. 2048.* – Women Development Democracy A study of Socio-Economic Changes in the Status of Women in Nepal.- (1981 – 1993).

Pradhan G. (1996) *Back Home From Brothels.* Kathlmandu: CWIN.

Rape for Profit Trafficking of Nepali Girls and Women to India's Brothels. (1995) New York: Human Rights Watch Asia.

Red Light Traffic (1996) Kathmandu: ABC- Nepal.

12. FOREIGN INTERVENTION IN POLITICS THROUGH NGOS: A CASE OF THE LEFT IN NEPAL

Gopal Siwakoti 'Chintan'

INTRODUCTION

In the past, there were a good number of Nepali movements working against Indian hegemonic and Western capitalist sentiments. However, they were not very successful since the political parties and other social movements were forced to operate underground during the past Panchayati regime. Moreover, foreigners were trying to control and suppress these movements for their interests.

At the same time, the Palace was attracted to the foreign resources that NGOs could bring and to the political control that could be imposed on those resources. Before 1990, Her Majesty the Queen was the chairperson of the then Social Service National Coordination Council. Foreigners were not allowed free access to every sector of society. There was some control of the NGO sector, and they were also tightly controlled by the Palace which was using NGOs for its own interest.

However, things have become very different since the establishment of an open society in 1990. Organizations can be established without restrictions or limitations. Anyone can do anything in any party of the country which is facilitated by lack of appropriate legal and administrative control. In fact, the people who are supposed the run the government, such as Members of Parliament and government officials, themselves are involved directly or indirectly in the operation of NGOs for personal gains. They have been efficient in mobilizing outside resources due to their easy access to and influence on the donors. They started operating NGOs in the name of their family members and relatives. They also started earning much more through the NGOs than from the public offices.

Unfortunately, there has not been sufficient control over this conflict of interests. In these situations, the foreigners and the donors worked closely with these public figures and the government officials through their money and projects, and became successful in preparing project or policy reports of their choice and priority. It became a powerful tool of penetrating into Nepali political leadership and the decision-makers leading to the replacement of our good government programs and policies by the bad ones. The easy financial gain, and opportunities to travel abroad or having their children attend the best colleges and universities in the West have contributed mightily to the weakening of national identity. The political parties and the bureaucracy, in effect, became easily accessible to foreign influences lending to significant abuse.

In short, foreigners and donors have often pursued their own agenda, at the high cost of supplanting long standing policies and beliefs of our own. It has evolved into an unfortunate situation where the Nepali people govern in favor of foreign interests rather than in the interests of their own people, systematically allowing foreign influence and penetration, and dismantle our indigenous state/social structures and infrastructures.

Today, it is possible for foreigners/donors to do nearly anything they want through the manipulation of the governmental system, including the judiciary, in the name of legal/judicial reforms in the interest of multinational companies. The process of policy and institutional change in the past few years have become rapid and rampant. The consequences of foreign intervention/penetration through the process of NGOization of local political and social movements include: (1) the gradual loss of our national policies, programs and priorities; (2) the nature of laws enacted by the Parliament in favor of foreign interests, formulation of new policies and programs against the spirit and the objectives of the Constitution; (3) forcing the country towards the imperialist economic globalisation, gradual privatization of public/social sectors, e.g. drinking water, electricity, telecommunications, education, health, agriculture and food; and (4) the foreignization and multicorporatization of public corporations and social services in the name of privation against national and public interest. It has shown in the past that there is nothing much that can do done by any political party even if it joins the government since the hands of the policy-makers and the bureaucrats are already tied, and, they also have been doing it knowingly under the pressure of foreign powers and agencies. This has made Nepal's political and economic future more and more difficult even for the upcoming generations. To say the least, the country is going to face severe consequences of this disaster.

At the same, in the field of NGOs, the most severe loss has been the NGOization of political parties. It is an unrecoverable loss for Nepal to have her leaders, particularly those of Marxist and Leninist belief, to fall knowingly into the trap of the same Western economic interest that they are philosophically and ideologically supposed to oppose. We may have to wait for several decades to recover from this loss.

REASONS BEHIND THE MUSHROOMING GROWTH OF NGOS

First of all, we have to make a distinction between non-governmental organizations (NGOs) and people-based movements. NGOs are generally known as those formed by a few individuals or their family members with specific objectives of providing service or doing some development work in the local area. Movements, on the other hand, are people-based organizations, organized with certain political objectives, and as far as possible, based on a particular class ideology, or promoting the rights of women, peasants, labors, workers, and indigenous peoples. Similarly, those organizations established to raise awareness and generate public pressure in the field of human rights, environmental protection and people-centered development are also known as movements.

At international level, generally, all organizations working outside the government periphery are put in one category as NGOs. In the case of Nepal, NGOs are known as those established as desired by the foreigners or for the purpose of having easy access to foreign money or use that fund for political party workers or their organizational expansion or influencing the voters during elections.

In this context, we can say that there were hardly any NGOs like we have today until the restoration of multi-party system in 1990. The point is that there were more campaigns and movements, and not NGOs, during the Panchayati regime. The activities used to take place at peoples' level and all necessary resources used to be collected from the people. NGOs were not used as a begging bowl or an employment agency. Foreigners had no chance of infiltration. As a result, the Nepali people were able to launch the 1990 Peoples' Movement that restored multi-party system. The people of Nepal were successful to achieve certain freedoms, although they are limited, and stimulate a feeling of change.

Before 1990 there were movements of the people in different sectors, such as patriotic, leftist and progressive movements, and they were gaining strength. The main objectives of all these movements were to oppose exploitation and repression, Indian hegemonies and Western imperialism, the growing expansion of Western monopoly capitalism, free-market economy and privatization leading to economic imperialism and neo-colonialism. However, today these campaigns and movements, with some exceptions, have been converted into NGOs. Their attitude and working style has been dominated by NGO-culture. Their activities cannot be sustained without foreign funds. Even people with a good track record and political commitment such as intellectuals and academics have become part of NGOism leading to a great loss for the nation. Moreover, NGO-culture is giving birth to a new and highly luxurious and corrupt class of people. It is diverting the strength of youth away from socio-political and anti-imperialist movements. The people who could be the leaders in these movements are running away with excuses of political corruption, poverty and unemployment. They have been smart enough to define NGOs as parallel to social work, and that NGOs offer them name, fame, wealth, and even political gain. This has been spreading all over the country as a chronic disease. The process of mushrooming of NGOs as well as their death is also rampant.

FOREIGN INTERVENTION IN NEPALI POLITICS THROUGH NGOS

The foreign intervention in Nepali politics through NGOs can be understood in two forms: (1) infiltration and undue influence in internal political organization and their decision-making process; and (2) theoretical penetration through misinterpretation of their political philosophy, ideology, fundamental policies and principles in the name of searching alternatives to political adjustment in the so called contemporary anti-communist world.

a) Political/Organizational Intervention/Penetration

It is a grand design and global strategy of imperialist and anti-left Western countries to penetrate Nepal's most powerful and influential leftist political parties and destroy them from within. It is not a surprise for us to know that there has been a headache in the growth of Nepali left movement, and the Western powers are "celebrating" the "death" of socialism in the world. We can easily understand this scenario, for example, in the case of Nepal, where the United States during the Peoples' Movement in 1990 was giving all the political support to the then Panchayati regime and the Palace, and was the first country to immediately make a public statement in support of the multi-party system once it was restored.

The western donors do not support organizations or individuals who oppose globalisation, free market economy, economic liberalization and privatization. Their support is geared to increase their own influence and expand the global market, and not to work in the interest of Nepal and the Nepali people. There are a few donors who are liberal but they have not been very influential.

Today, these international institutions, donor countries and international non-governmental organizations (INGOs) have been directly reaching at local levels throughout the country but the local efforts are often undermined because local leaders are enticed by foreign influence and willing to conform to whatever these INGOs propose. To compound the problem, these local leaders often express frustration toward their own political parties and government agencies which have so far failed to address basic problems in their respective communities. In terms of the foreign influence, the INGOs encourage them to register and to have their own NGOs. They provide them money for sometime. They create illusions about politics or ask them to be engaged in NGO work by maintaining their party links. This makes these local leaders more wealthy all of a sudden and they become habituated to what they use to avoid before. S/he becomes dependent economically and in material terms from foreign agency. At the same time, s/he also maintains his/her link with the party intact. S/he supports financially to his/her party leaders close to him/her, offers good food, arranges foreign travel and/or conducts NGO activities in the electoral constituency of the leaders or of his/her own relatives who may be running for elections for the parliament or local bodies. These NGO activities include drilling tub-well, distributing sewing machines, medicines and running micro-credit programs and other projects. By this time, a full-time political party worker becomes a powerful NGO worker with more influence over his party and the leaders.

Unfortunately, many parties with long history of political struggle have turned to NGOs for support. Parties find it difficult to function and win election successfully without NGO workers, their funds and local projects. For the left parties this has meant that they cannot talk anymore about revolution or total change and they can no longer oppose the economic and social policies and programs or the big and destructive development projects. If it does anything contrary, then it loses all the donor support that it is now dependent on. If the same thing is done by the party-affiliated NGO worker, s/he loses his/her social status and appeal because s/he does not receive the same amount of money as before. S/he becomes helpless and decides to sacrifice all his/her party, ideology, patriotism and the revolutionary goals. His/her NGO becomes a tool of the West and they all become their permanent servants. And, ultimately, the donors close down their projects after turning all the best political cadres and social workers into typical NGO workers, and away from political struggles. In this stage, there would be neither NGOs nor political movement or campaign in this country. This is how countries like Nepal are converted into the monopoly market of the West from society to consumer goods. They turn the people and the country economically dependent and mentally as their servants.

There was a time when no members of the communist organizations were permitted to visit the United States. But, through NGOs, they were able to travel from Europe to North America and elsewhere. They gradually started thinking that NGO is the better choice than to run a revolutionary party, to become a Member of Parliament or to look for opportunities and gains in the government since NGOs can be used for easy access to foreign fund and financial gain, foreign travel, projects in electoral constituencies. It became easier for them to win elections through NGO activities by influencing the voters through varieties of little projects here and there, and by conducting NGO orientation classes instead of political teaching. They thought that doing development work through NGOs was much more easy and quick to satisfy the voters than the dream of an elected government or a revolution. As a result, the high-command brains of the party began to devote their valuable time and energy into NGO competition. They started wasting all their strength in managing NGOs instead of running the party, leading the mass movements and launching other campaigns. They even started taking direct or indirect actions against those who failed to provide financial support to the party as a kind of 'levy', and they further adopted the policy of non-cooperation to those failing the party line in the NGO management. Even human rights groups and the social movements are not free from this tragedy. In recent years, there have been so many incidents of NGO capture, manipulation and character assassination of activists and division among themselves. It is ultimately killing the roots of the human rights, environmental and social movements. There are cases in which independent human rights groups and organizations are struggling very hard for their integrity and independence from political parties.

Therefore, despite the fact that around thirty-thousands NGOs were established in Nepal in one decade, the country is losing the very basic nature and character of the movement, mass-based actions and campaigns. NGO network and their financial capacity has become critical for many political party candidates to win elections in the Parliament or in the local bodies. However, the bitter reality is that most of these NGOs and the highly sophisticated political parties cannot run or function in the same manner as they are now if the foreign fund is to be suspended, let us say, just for a period of six months. They will crumble like castles of sand. This will have very serious impacts for political parties like Communist Party of Nepal - United Marxist-Leninist (CPN-UML) and, the other so called high-profile NGOs and NGO-sponsored human rights groups in town. It is really very unfortunate that our proletarian leaders have now become the 'special citizens' of the country with Pajero, luxurious buildings, foreign wine. They have their children studying in the West or other best schools in Nepal or other neighboring countries. Their past sacrifice has been wasted, and thus, has no value! In short, the people of Nepal are lose great revolutionary leaders of their time. They may have to work again for an indefinite period of time to give a birth to a new party and leaders. Even in the case of CPN-UML, there is nothing to be happy about, only regret. It is now not difficult to reach the conclusion that there are millionaires in the NGO market with all kinds access to power and politics. Some NGOs and INGOs have their own network all over the country which is parallel to the party. It is also not difficult to identify who is doing what, how and for whom, including their involvement in the criminalization of political and the corruption of politicians. There is a need of thorough research and analysis to expose them to the public. It is also important to know about those groups who collect data from police department or collect information about local events and incidents, like rape or accident, and compile as the reports of human rights violations. It is misleading the people and the very core of the human rights movement.

On the other hand, the Western donors are investing more and more energy where the anti-imperialist, patriotic and the left movement is strong. They are presenting NGOs as the 'only' and the 'best' alternatives to any movements or revolution. In most of the countries, they have been very successful in misleading the movement and the people. For them, it is always worth investing millions to NGOs than to invest billions in arms and other diplomatic waste for the suppression of the movement or topple down a revolutionary government. And, it is much more easier and sophisticated if it is done through NGOs in which they also become the 'donor' and the 'sole decision-maker'. The Westerners and the donors have been successful to dilute the Nepal's mass-based democratic-leftist movement just in one decade without any arms-sale or war, simply by spending a couple of millions and defame our leaders. Now, the leaders and the Members of Parliament cannot hardly visit their own constituencies without an NGO or a project. At the same time, they are developing the attitude and inferiority complex of not being able to win elections, form a government and do any development work without the support of India or Western imperialist economic power; and, the financial and trade institutions such as the World Bank, IMF and WTO. Foreign interest is highly visible in all governmental sectors and at decision-making levels, further hindering change in the best interest of our people.

One typical example is the involvement of USAID, the Asia Foundation and the National Democratic Institute (NDI) in Nepal's parliamentary exercise and democratization process. Our leaders are being manipulated and as treated as their servants, thinking that they cannot do anything in the Parliament or in the government without having lunch and dinner with these so called experts of 'democracy' and 'human rights' in five star hotels or without attending their orientation training or visits in the West during their parliamentary sessions and elections. They are now even taking training from the under-graduate level experts of democracy coming from the United States on how to organize a meeting, give a speech and write a paper submitted to the Parliament. It is most unfortunate for Nepal and the Nepali people. It shows that our one-time revolutionary leaders are not even fit for the parliamentary politics without foreign support such as USAID and NDI.

b) Theoretical penetration

The second type of foreign penetration is in political theory and ideology that we Nepalis believe in. In the first place, they already have developed the attitude of economic dependence in all governmental function, and the so called development work that foreign aid and loan is the alternative for our survival. This is a total mental bankruptcy. So, almost all our mainstream political parties and leaders, both from 'right' to the 'left' or others have accepted and adopted the policy and package of Western monopoly free-market economy, globalisation, Structural Adjustment Program (SAP), and promotion of large and destructive dams constructed by multinational companies. It is so visible in the recent election manifestos of Nepal's major political parties. They lack vision, perspectives and plans for the country. NGOs have been used as influential tool in this destructive brain-washing and Western ideological indoctrination against the country's priorities and the peoples' movement.

The saddest part of all this is that the NGOs or so called labor or women's organizations are silent about these issues that their leaders have believed in, and even if they say something about it, it is typically for the sake of formality or to gain support. The very simple reason is that they do not get any money to do these critical things from the donors. For example, in the case of the landmark campaign against the World Bank-managed Arun III Hydroelectric Project (which was canceled in 1995 after two years of campaign and opposition to it), the supporters and cadres of the CPN-UML tried to hijack the campaign and take over the Arun Concerned Group (the Arun III campaign network) once the CPN-UML formed the government and decided to accept the Arun III Project in its original form. There are so many national issues of concerns that are demanding high-level campaigns in the country in recent years from water resources and environmental destruction to the signing by Nepal of different bi-lateral and multi-lateral treaties that are against the interests of the people and the country.

ALTERNATIVES AND CONCLUSIONS

Finally, the above analysis does not suggest that all NGOs are bad and that all the work that they are doing is not helpful at all. But, in the case of Nepal, we are talking about an extreme scenario of NGOs. We are talking about the attempt of NGOs to take over the role of the State, dilute and destroy the democratic and social movement, increasing dependency everywhere and inviting, knowingly or unknowingly, the Western/foreign vested political and economic interests in the country. They have been misused or being compromised against the interests of the people and the movements for their narrow financial gain, greed and luxury. As a result, these are not only NGOs themselves, but the whole human rights and social movements are gradually loosing their credibility and faith from among the people at the hands of the NGO culture. Of paramount importance thus, is addressing how to control and prevent their presence and influence in the political parties and the process. Otherwise, Nepal's political, social and human rights movements will be endangered in such a way that nothing can be done without foreign support. The left, particularly, will be destroyed for a long period of time. In such situation, no one in Nepal will be in a position to achieve and guarantee economic, social, political, cultural and developmental rights to the Nepali people. It has been difficult to fight against Indian hegemonism, US imperialism and other Western capitalist countries.

Therefore, our need today is not of NGOs or their projects, but of process and a real change with content. All the work that NGOs claim to do can be done more easily and more effectively by the local government bodies (i.e., 4000 Village Development Committees, 60 municipalities, and 75 District Development Committees as well as other local and community based consumer/pressure groups). It is also their duty and responsibility according to the law as well as to the commitment to the people. The primary obstacle is controlling the resources that are now being grossly misused and wasted by these unaccountable NGOs mostly based in Kathmandu, and using these same resources in making our politicians and the political process as corrupt and unethical, including political criminalization. Obtaining the resources would be more than enough to implement all the plans and priorities that we have in the country for decades in all parts of Nepal. The dilemma is NGOs have money but no vision, no plans, inadequate capacity and no mandate. On the other hand, the real State agencies and local bodies have all the vision, plans, capacity and the mandate, but no resources. It is just not fair.

However, it does not mean that the problems are only NGOs and the donors/foreigners. Our leaders, bureaucrats and the people are also responsible for it. We can see in their manifestos that they would like to strengthen the capacity of NGOs and involve them actively in developmental activities. It is very inappropriate and useless. If NGOs are the solutions then why do we need political parties based on different political and economic ideologies, and why do we need a State or a government or Parliament and why do we need elections? Why not give all the responsibility for national building to the NGOs and donors? Because it will be totally wrong, and we should never allow it to happen.

Finally, the following urgent measures can be discussed as part of recommendations to prevent and control foreign intervention/penetration in the internal politics of Nepal:

- All the external resources have to be centrally coordinated and utilized/decentralized for the local bodies and the community-based consumer groups based on our local and national priorities and needs. All the resources must reach all the way down to the target areas. Any NGOs or INGOs or the donors have to be prevented from developing and implementing any projects of their own, including the setting of priority according to their interests. They have to be asked to disclose all the sources and amounts of funds that they have and the types of activities/sectors/areas that they would like fund and the reasons behind it, including the compliance with our local and national priorities. They have to pay taxes. Otherwise, we will not be solving any problems just on the basis of how much money (and sometime even more money than it is actually needed) that we bring in the name child labor, bonded labor, girls/women trafficking and so on. In my view, many NGOs/INGOs have become part of the problems rather than a solution.

- No projects should be allowed to run by any member of a political party or any elected officials or leaders or Members of Parliament or government officials and/or their close relatives other than advocacy and awareness-raising.

- We have to be able to create strong public opinion against those who misuse their organizations and their objectives and destroy or undermine the social movements and human rights campaigns, particularly those who are running NGOs under the direct or indirect banner of a particular political party.

- All activities of the donors and the foreigners have to be closely monitored and the government has to develop a mechanism to decide whether a particular donor or an INGO should be allowed to work and how and where. There has to be clear and strongly policy as in the case of other donor countries as well. They have to be expelled when their activities are found against the social, political and economic interest of Nepal and the Nepali people.

- There should be no provision for the transaction of foreign currency by NGOs or any groups or agencies operating outside the government and without the knowledge of the government. A separate but efficient mechanism has to be developed to coordinate such activities and facilitate the work of good NGOs which mobilize internal or external resources and direct involve local constituents and the local government bodies.

In conclusion, it is better not to have any NGOs rather than to have them style and form that they exist and operate now. There would be no additional damage or loss to the people or the communities. It will not further deteriorate the economic situation or social conditions of the poverty-driven majority of the Nepali people. It has already gotten far worse than one could imagine. The country has gone down with almost no point of return. NGOs have become mostly dependent, and they have become more donors-oriented rather than their own people. To allow NGOs up to the level of having too much influence in the political parties is a very destructive and anti-people work. Therefore, the government of Nepal, the political parties and the people of Nepal have to be alert to develop new thoughts about the role of NGOs and the donors as well as finding alternatives for them and their work.

Box 1.

COMMUNITY FORESTRY MOVEMENT AND VOLUNTARY ORGANISATIONS IN NEPAL

Narayan Kaji Shrestha

In Nepal there are some 8000 forest areas formally controlled by community forestry user groups, and equal number may be done informally. According to the former Secretary of Forests and soil Conservation "Wherever you see green and living forests they are managed by users, and wherever you see depleting and dead forests they are supposed to be managed by the government". This has been a major achievement after decades of centralised control for the benefit of the elites.

However, there are some fears and dangers looming. Elites and powerful are gradually taking control of the decision making by marginalising poor, disadvantaged and women in the community forests. National and international companies are eyeing for concessions and putting pressures on the government and users. Very influential and greedy group of bureaucrats and politicians still want to use forest for their benefits by disempowering people and even by changing policy. People's success and honest attempts are not highlighted but a few and small human mistakes by users are trumpeted. In spite of the proven fact that forest bureaucracy is not a capable and efficient institution, it wants to assert its rights over forest resources in the name of the Operational Forest Management Plan. Most surprising fact is that the donors push this idea. This has led to confusion and blocked the community forestry campaign and local people's aspirations for managing own resources and bringing positive changes and development in their own communities.

The voluntary sector in Nepal for certain reasons have not been that actively engaged in community forestry campaign in spite that this is a very potential sector for them to contribute. Only a very few INGOs and NGOs are involved with somewhat seriousness. In terms of participatory process and empowerment, voluntary sectors can learn a lot from the Community Forestry campaign.

Basically, there are four pillars involved in the community forest: government forest agency, donors, users and voluntary agencies. Usually, the forest agencies and donors will cooperate and work together because of compulsion. Users are joining hands and building alliances under the Federation of Community Forest Users, Nepal (FECOFUN). However, the FECOFUN is quite handicapped in their struggle with the highly educated, equipped and resourceful entities. Voluntary organisations (VO) can support and be an ally with the FECOFUN in this struggle. Ultimately, people will win but support from the VOs enhance capacity of users and boost their moralities.

Let's lock at an example: by policy 61% forest is supposed to come under user group forestry. Out of 5.5 million ha of forests in Nepal, two million are National Parks, Protected Areas and Reserves. Similarly, a few thousand ha come under the buffer zone management, so remaining forest is, in fact, less than 61%. However, the Department of Forests is shying away to hand over such remaining forests, rather they are coming up with idea of the Operational Forest Management Plan (OFMP), which empowers them to take over forests allocated as community forests. As forest handing-over process is hampered with such an excuse especially in the Terai region, FECOFUN has started to raise this issue. However, the government agencies do not feel need for responding. This is a case where the VOs can play very critical role in terms of raising awareness and lobbying with users. Also, if users are managing resources properly, why is there hesitation to hand over the forests to communities? VOs can raise such question more forcefully and effectively. In the name of the dreaded OFMP, forest officials have started marking trees for harvest but by visiting such forests it is clear that it is not any scientific management but marking of any marketable and exportable tree. Probably, VOs can help raise awareness of local users about their rights, organise them for their rights, lobby and expose such practices up to national and international level as and when required.

Community forests are gradually being controlled by elites and powerful again because of proper processes are not being followed before handing over. Some cynics see this as a design to make CF unsuccessful. People need to be made aware of their rights, empowered to make own decisions, help them come to consensus, and have confidence to trust their knowledge, skills and decisions. Here, VOs as champions of organising and empowering communities have opportunity to help and support users.

Right now, community forests can be divided equally into three types. First, chairman's forest, second, committee's forest and, third, communities' forest. There is need for reformulating former two kinds into real community forest, otherwise they will be bad examples of community forests which might provide even ammunitions for quashing the community forestry campaign. Here again, VOs can play critical role. The Terai Community Forestry Action Team, an alliance of 13 I/NGOs have been playing such role in the Terai area which can be expanded to the Hills also.

User managed forest resources are generating fund which are being used for some community development activities but 80/90% of such fund are lying idle. VOs can help user groups plan for use of such fund, build capacity to manage, and develop required skills. In fact, it will help VOs to extricate themselves from clutches of donors and their unexplainable demands and requirements, which means they may be able to become real voluntary organisations rather than imposed and directed by external agencies.

Dr. Narayan Kaji Shresta is associated with Kathmandu based women's organisation WATCH.

PART III EXPERIENCES FROM ELSEWHERE IN SOUTH ASIA

13. ENABLING THE DISABILITY NGOS? CENTRALISATION VERSUS COMPETITION IN PAKISTAN AND BANGLADESH

M. Miles

INTRODUCTION

This chapter reviews contrasting patterns of 'Disability NGO' development in Pakistan and Bangladesh, two nations with some political, cultural and socio-economic similarities. After sketching the historical background, the focus will be on mental retardation (MR) service organisations from the early 1980s to mid 1990s, a period during which those NGOs expanded, mostly with foreign assistance. In Pakistan several small, autonomous NGOs worked locally and provincially, often centred on particular schools or service units. Some practical collaboration took place, but the NGOs were often in mutual competition for resources and kudos. As the number of NGOs increased, repeated efforts were made to achieve a Pakistan-wide platform and co-ordination, but geographical factors and friction between various participating groups and viewpoints prevented any lasting success. In Bangladesh, centralisation of power took place very early in the development process, under a single national MR organisation which then spread its branches across the country, heavily supported by Nordic aid; yet this monopoly was also challenged, allowing a variety of grassroots responses to MR. Comparison of the divergent development patterns in Pakistan and Bangladesh is difficult because of the many unmeasurable factors. Nevertheless, some experiences common to the NGOs in both countries suggest that neither development pattern is inherently superior.

WELFARE NGOS IN SOUTH ASIAN HISTORY

The literature of South Asian antiquity provides fascinating but inconclusive glimpses of a range of individual and communal practices in welfare assistance to disabled people[1]. Best known are the centralised arrangements whereby the ruler of a city or region was responsible for providing food and shelter to 'the sick, the lame, the blind', either permanently or by special arrangement during famines or natural catastrophes. Thus Draupadi, the archetypal wife of the Pandavas, was seen daily serving all her company "including even the deformed and the dwarfs"

---

[1] These and some later aspects of NGO work in South Asia are documented and discussed in detail in Miles (1999, chapters 2, 6, 7 and 8). Versions of chapters 7 and 8 have appeared also in Miles (1998a, 1998b).

(Mahabharata, Sabha Parva 51). In various Ramayana versions, employment of hunchbacked servants at court reflected an apparently widespread practice. Yet the traditional celebration of philanthropy by the nobility may divert attention from the ordinary householder obligation to provide for the needy person who begged food at the door, a duty enjoined from Vedic times and perhaps responsible for a much wider charitable support to disabled people than any courtly efforts.

Somewhere between the court and the individual household there were indications of 'civil society' in the self-organised groups that undertook socially beneficial activities of their own choosing. Some Jataka stories suggest that groups of families or maybe a whole street of householders, or a trade guild, might act together to feed needy people. From early Buddhist and Jaina sources two further long-lasting traditions emerged. One was the community-supported monastic practice of giving asylum to some disabled children who then grew up with a religious education and some practical skills, such as music-making, by which they might become self-supporting. In sharp contrast were the practices embodied in the strangely modern sounding legend of Manimekhalai, the pretty young social worker with a high media profile, surrounded by a throng of blind, lame, decrepit and hungry people on whom she scattered her semi-organised beneficence (Dani, lou & Gopala Ayer 1993). The rise of Muslim power particularly across North India seems to have made little practical difference to the various traditional forms of charity. Some Muslim rulers created charitable institutions, while Muslim communities had their bait-ul-mal or community chest for relieving poverty and their auqaf trusts for perpetuating benevolence (or for avoiding taxation) (Rashid 1978; Kozlowski 1995). Certain occupations became the preserve of blind men, e.g. memorising and declaiming the Qur'an, while deaf men traditionally became tailors. The small numbers of Europeans arriving from the 16th century also made little difference during their first two centuries, as they slowly developed measures to care for their own disabled or needy people.

NGO welfare activities on a larger scale can be documented from early 19th century Bengal onward. Growing numbers of British merchants, soldiers and East India Company officials consolidating their grip on ever larger parts of North India began to discover that governmental power secured 'for the purpose of trade' could not altogether be divorced from the welfare obligations traditionally associated with rulers. Printing presses were increasingly used to create and mould public (i.e. literate) opinion among both European and Indian educated classes, and to highlight moral demands upon them, an essential ingredient for the nascent conscience of civil society. NGOs to promote education and welfare began with Europeans in charge and some wealthy Indian collaborators, but within a few years the balance shifted and Indians created their own NGOs for a wide range of social purposes.[2] NGOs benefiting disabled people originated probably in the 1810s with public efforts to start a leprosy asylum at Calcutta. A longer-lasting initiative was the opening of Raja Kali Shankar Ghosal's Blind Asylum at Benares in 1826, involving the Raja as a concerned individual, his researchers who enumerated the local blind people, a group of British officials as trustees, some East India Company funds, some private and civic subscriptions, many people subsequently taking an interest in the blind residents, and eventually some special educational provisions in the 1860s by European missionaries. In these activities at Benares no single modern-style constitutional NGO is clearly identifiable, yet a range of charitable and educational actions occurred that were done neither by an individual nor by government, but by community action.

Nineteenth century India also saw some trends and movements that slowly generated knowledge about child learning and development, kindergartens, progressive pedagogy and legal measures concerned with mental incapacity. An 'Idiot Asylum' flourished in the 1840s and 1850s at Madras, in which experience was gained of occupational therapy with mentally retarded people. The first half of the 20th century added the development of psychological testing, measurements of mental abilities, school health services, formal classes for 'idiots' in mental hospitals, and a growing concern for children who attended ordinary schools but who learnt very slowly if at all (Miles 1998a; 1998b). It was not until the 1960s, however, that parental concerns for such children extended beyond the privacy of the family and issued in NGOs that would battle in the public arena. By this period, there had already been much more substantial experience of concerted South Asian voluntary welfare action, as for example by the Arya Samaj and the Ramakrishna Mission, followed by Gokhale's Servants of India Society, the Bengal Social Service League, Gandhi's paternalistic Harijan Sevak Sangh, and the grassroots efforts of Co-operative Societies (Strickland 1939, especially pp. 317-340, 380-392). The possibilities of large NGOs with centralised power acting through dispersed branches, as against small, locally responsive NGOs acting in loose-knit confederations, were recognised as alternative development paths in the earlier 20th century.

---

[2] Some of the wealthier Indians, after studying the psychology of their foreign rulers, could afford to give the latter a few public lessons in humility. The British could be upstaged simply by colossal donations, as when "Dwarakanath Tagore made a startling announcement of a big donation of Rs.100,000 to the [District Charitable] Society in 1838. ... The Europeans were naturally stunned, and so were the Indians." (Sanyal 1977, 105-106). Still more pointed was the "Hospital for poor Europeans" erected by Babu Guru Das Mittra, a Bengali leader at Benares (Sherring 1875, p.82) Wealthy Indian businessmen tended to avoid all such ironies and were assiduous supporters of 'progressive' British-led charities; yet simultaneously they supported traditional charitable approaches of the sort that the British reformers were trying to replace (Haynes 1987).

NGO DEVELOPMENTS IN PAKISTAN

The first NGOs concerned with MR in Pakistan were initiated very largely by fathers having a mentally retarded child, in collaboration with a few other concerned people. This repeated the pattern of an earlier movement by parents of deaf children in the 1940s to press for services, which resulted in the formation of a 'Deaf and Dumb Welfare Society' at Lahore in 1949, followed by the opening of a special school (Makhdum 1961, 6-7). The first MR pioneer, Mr A. S. Muslim, began in classic fashion with a letter in the major Urdu and English newspapers in 1959, stating that he had a mentally retarded child and did not know where to find help. Replies poured in from far and near, and in 1960 he founded SCINOSA, the Society for Children in Need of Special Attention, with an elected governing body of two physicians, a lawyer, a social worker, a retired senior civil servant and a businessman, three of them being fathers of disabled children. Muslim has described with some bitterness the lack of interest or attempted dissuasion from some senior professionals whom he consulted in Karachi. He took encouragement from seeing a centre at Bombay run by Mrs. Jai Vakeel, who later provided the constitution of her society as a model for SCINOSA. Eventually Muslim patterned his activities on work that he visited during a business trip to Norway, and in 1962 a similar day centre was opened at Karachi for his own son and others like him. SCINOSA started with practically no funds, equipment or accommodation, but Muslim and his co-workers begged here and there for cash and volunteer help and meanwhile began daily work with the children who were the intended beneficiaries (Muslim 1993, 58-89). The actual schooling was amateurish at the start, but staff gained experience as they went along and some ideas and equipment were borrowed from the Montessori movement.

The Karachi experiences helped another parent of a mentally retarded child, West Pakistan's former Auditor-General Syed Yaqoob Shah, at Lahore. With others, he formed an NGO called the West Pakistan Society for the Welfare of Mentally Retarded Children, and the centre 'Amin Maktab' was opened in 1962, also with some difficulties (Pakistan Society 1993). In Pakistan's third major city, Mr Bhandara, who had a mentally retarded son and owned Pakistan's main brewery, was a leading figure in the third NGO to open a special school. Bhandara (1971) introduced the work as "a Society for Mentally Handicapped Children which was established in a small room in Satellite Town, Rawalpindi, by a devoted Social Worker Lady Miss Julia Riggs with the help and assistance of some Pakistani and Foreign ladies in Jan. 1970. A School under the auspices of the Society was subsequently started on a very small scale. ... At present there are about 20 children in the school." In addition to these schools or day-centres managed by small, local NGOs with a progressive, educational outlook, one residential institution was opened at Karachi in 1969 by a Dutch nun (whose own sister in the Netherlands had Down's syndrome) for children considered to have profound or multiple handicaps. This became the only place in Pakistan where several score of families could permanently deposit children with severe disabilities to be 'cared for'. A fifth initiative, in 1974, followed a slightly more complicated path. The Mental Health Centre (MHC), Peshawar, already existed as a psychiatric centre and a rural community mental health scheme, under the Church of Pakistan. An urban play-group was begun for mentally retarded children and their mothers, and this later became a school and resource centre. The Frontier Association for the Mentally Handicapped (FAMH) was set up to provide for membership and campaigning activities, without having a direct role in the play-group and later school, whether as fund-raising body or management committee, as the latter functions were undertaken by the MHC.

These early NGOs and subsequent ones went through a cumbersome process of formulating a constitution and getting themselves registered with the Provincial Department of Social Welfare, on a pattern derived from Societies Registration laws enacted by the British Indian government in the 1860s and scarcely changed since then. The provisions were intended to give a legal framework, some democratic checks and balances, a turn-over of officers by regular elections, and a closely controlled financial accountability. In practice the rules and regulations seemed poorly adapted to the actual situations of NGOs in the 1960s or subsequently. Some NGOs have ignored them completely, while others have spent time and ingenuity on complying with the absolute minimum of requirements. The conception of the model NGO constitution was, and still is, alien to the culture of Pakistan, in which the long traditions of charitable effort followed an Islamic pattern of predominantly individual and family benevolence rather than a group cooperative pattern (Stillman 1975). NGO constitutions tended to be noticed only when a quarrel had broken out and dissident members hired a lawyer and obtained a court order stopping all proceedings on the grounds that no proper elections had been held, no accounts produced, etc. A study of the functioning of NGOs in the North-West Frontier Province (of which Peshawar is the capital) considered that it was "a serious shortcoming of the voluntary welfare societies", that with a few exceptions they seemed to be "managed year in year out by the same persons irrespective of their organising ability", and that this monopolisation caused them to "look like private concerns", to the extent that people were "bound to become suspicious of their real purpose" (Khan 1972, 74). The observation was and is undoubtedly correct, and reflects a situation to be found in many countries. Whether it is a serious shortcoming of the NGOs, or merely a reflection of development realities, has not so clearly been demonstrated.

The present author, who ran the Mental Health Centre, Peshawar, from 1978 to 1990 and was the active officer of the FAMH throughout the same period, tried to comply with at least the minimum of constitutional requirements, keeping accounts, maintaining a list of paid-up members, notifying them of the

Annual General Meeting and elections etc. In practice however the active membership consisted of the same three or four people throughout the 1980s, and a small number of others consented to their names appearing as 'sleeping' officers. The active Pakistani participants, one being a senior lawyer, viewed with kindly amusement their foreign colleague's efforts to keep within the rules, which none of them took seriously. In the earlier years, the FAMH was 'sponsored' by the local Rotary Club, whose members co-operated whenever a formal meeting was legally required. Later, parents or close relatives of some 40- 45 children attending the MHC day school were deemed to be honorary FAMH members, the school fees being counted in lieu of their 'subscription'. This meant that a good attendance could be achieved at a public meeting (without resort to hiring students to pack the hall), but practically none of these people was actually a paid-up, voting member. The FAMH AGM was combined with a meeting of parents and MHC staff, held in a local college with grounds in which the children could play and quantities of food and drink could be eaten or spilt and trodden into the floor without serious damage. These events were much appreciated by parents and children, and occasionally an 'issue' was presented to them for a democratic expression of their views; but the biennial elections were held at a different time. The FAMH thus served as an artificial construction, having an identity and legal basis that was usefully separate from that of the MHC (the latter suffering the triple stigma of association with 'madness', with foreigners, and with the Church of Pakistan, most of whose members were from the poorest socio-economic stratum).

The very small active FAMH membership included two or three well-respected Muslim professionals, one being the father of a mentally retarded child, who understood the usefulness of maintaining separate fronts for different purposes. They also understood very well that if we were trying to mobilise substantial resources in order to develop innovative services for much larger numbers of disabled children, there was little to be gained by encouraging the public at large, or parents with a special concern for their own child, to join up and take control of the organisation. During the 1980s the Federal Government was trying to spend money on disabled children, and the FAMH could easily show the necessary documentation in order to receive a grant, whereas the structure of the MHC (which was largely funded from abroad) would have been more difficult to accommodate within official rules. One government grant resulted in the FAMH providing a vehicle and driver for pick and drop of some of the MHC school children, over many years, which meant that it could also prove that it was 'providing a service' to the expected beneficiaries.

A more substantial project run nominally under the FAMH, with the MHC school as resource centre and training base, was the FAMH / UNICEF Community Rehabilitation Development Project, which ran from 1982 to 1987 and mobilised people in ten other large Frontier towns and cities (populations between 40,000 and 150,000) to form locally autonomous NGOs to start some work of their own choosing, in their own town and vicinity, for the benefit of disabled children. The usual expectation would have been for the FAMH, as the provincial 'parent body', to treat all these local associations as its branches, and to sit on top of the pyramid, enjoying power and controlling whatever finances could be raised. It could have been a wonderful little 'rehabilitation empire'; but our development experience from 1978-1982 suggested that the few local people who might be interested in this sort of voluntary work would do it with energy and devotion only if they were managing their own affairs and solving their own problems. Our theory was that local people were most likely to know, or to find out, answers to questions like: who and where were the disabled children in their town, what services should be provided for them, who were the influential people, how could some accommodation be found, what sources of funds might there be, who could be given some training and then employed in a little school, or physical therapy centre, or cottage industry training scheme? The only essential thing not available in these towns and cities was specialised knowledge of what to do with disabled children, in terms of special teaching, physical therapy, helping some of them into ordinary schools, providing assistive devices. For this, we made arrangements to give training at the MHC for several months, to young employees sent by the local NGOs created through the development project.

These new local NGOs were mobilised in various ways and functioned in different ways, but there was always a core of two or three people who really ran things. Some were a little more democratic than others, but the central people tended, understandably, to keep a close grip on whatever they achieved.[3] Some of them had a disabled child, some perhaps wanted the fame and kudos of being 'social workers', some were 'born organisers' and were already running other community activities to which a little disability work was an attractive new feature. The UNICEF office, which was understaffed and in permanent crisis, introduced a different motivation when it gave out vehicles and physiotherapy equipment to some of the local leaders. The original idea had been that the vehicles' purposes and usage should be closely controlled; but UNICEF was not a development agency and gave little thought to the effects of its bounty - the overriding duty was simply to spend its budget each year, regardless of after-effects. The Federal Government was also keen to bestow funds on these new, small NGOs, because General Zia ul Haq, himself the father of a disabled child, wanted something done for disabled people while he was in power. Some Federal grants were well directed, others were inadvertently destructive. A grant of Rs.100,000/-, not a small sum in the 1980s, intended to encourage a hard-

---

[3] One who had visited families, collected money and worked hard to start a small school, but did not keep a tight grip on the reins, suffered an attempted 'election ambush'. A small group, wishing to harvest the fruit of this man's hard work, paid the small membership subscriptions to enrol 30 students, who would vote them onto the controlling committee.

working disability NGO in one town, accidentally went to a moribund NGO with a corrupt secretary in a town of a similar-sounding name. Two years later, both NGOs had ceased to function. It was a curious period, in which various INGOs and governments were desperate to spend money on disabled people, short of taking it out in bags and giving it to beggars in the bazar; but the NGO capacity to absorb money quickly and use it to develop appropriate services hardly matched the available cash. By the time the skills and capacity had developed, of course the bonanza had ended. The MHC's role as a resource and mobilisation centre, providing training, information and encouragement, severely stretched its capacities; yet at least the newer NGOs came to understand that the responsibility for success or failure in their own town really depended on their own efforts. Eventually, they were able to think about helping one another, and even going out to the surrounding rural areas (Peters & Rehman 1988).

Across Pakistan more NGOs concerned with MR emerged during the 1980s, mostly running a special school or centre. From six NGOs at the end of the 1970s, there were around thirty by 1990. Among these, three or four, like the FAMH, had a province-wide 'reach' and were strong enough to arrange conferences or training activity which others across the country could attend. From the mid-1980s onward, various efforts have been made to create a national forum that could speak with one voice and represent MR concerns to the government. For various reasons, none of these efforts succeeded. The geography of Pakistan is such that the mega-city of Karachi, with nearly half of the MR services, is separated from the heavily populated Punjab by several hundred miles of near-desert. MR activists in the North West Frontier and the Punjab could meet together at Lahore or Islamabad without excessive expense, but were reluctant to make the long trip to Karachi unless an airfare was provided. Karachi activists were unwilling to visit the north at their own expense. Only the Federal Government had sufficient funds to pay for a national meeting - but when it did so, naturally it had its own agenda and was not particularly concerned to foster a national MR organisation (which would certainly come with heavy demands for ongoing budgets, without providing disabled people with any direct services of the sort that create goodwill for the government).

Furthermore, for years the major MR NGOs had been in competition with one another for funding, trained staff, foreign assistance, and the image of being angels of mercy. Most of the key players could co-operate with one another at the occasional Federal Government meeting, but underneath there was a heavy backlog of mistrust and suspicion, sometimes exacerbated by parent / professional differences of viewpoint, sometimes by psychiatrist / psychologist differences, and other such irritants. Several major NGOs had taken up associate membership of the International League of Societies for the Mentally Handicapped, but none could achieve full membership with voting rights because that was available only to 'national' organisations. One Karachi NGO was a member of the Asian Federation for the Mentally Retarded and exclusively 'represented' Pakistan at the biennial meeting of this Federation. The foreign trips, competition for kudos and rumours of huge grants acquired from gullible foreign organisations, militated against co-operative activities and policy inputs on the national level. These various factors probably also reduced the effectiveness of all the NGOs in serving and advocating on behalf of mentally retarded people. However, it is not easy to prove any of these disadvantages. To have room and freedom to run one's own show, and to do so with some element of competitiveness, are powerful motivating factors. There is also more accumulation of experience and consistency of policy in NGOs that are run for many years by the same people, as compared with the sometimes rapid turnover of officers in more 'democratic' systems.

The best balance between new blood with fresh ideas, and old hands with solid experience, is seldom easy to achieve. No doubt the leaders of disability service NGOs ought to be saints with the purest motives and endless energy. In real life they / we seldom achieve sainthood, but are more likely to burn out and become difficult and demanding, while resenting and obstructing the work of the next generation of activists. It is perhaps enough if an NGO can achieve some development of resources, some activities, some education, some public awareness, where there was none before; and can demonstrate on the small scale some patterns of service development that invite government incorporation on a national scale. The achievement of such modest goals by Pakistan's MR NGOs was slowly but increasingly observable between 1960 and the mid-1990s. By the late 1980s the Federal Government had indeed adopted some of the approaches pioneered by NGOs, so that government officers have begun to build up their own experience of service provision, along with channels for parent participation. Foreign aid (and interference) played a significant part, with activity by VSO and the Peace Corps, British, American, German, Nordic, Japanese, Korean and Australian professionals and advisors, some overseas training, some import of equipment and methods. Perhaps the range and conflict of foreign viewpoints contributed to developing sophistication among Pakistani counterparts.[4]

NGO DEVELOPMENTS IN BANGLADESH

Many of the cultural features affecting NGOs in Pakistan have been equally reflected in Bangladesh, and will not here be repeated. From 1947 to 1961 East Pakistan experienced joint nationhood with West Pakistan, though separated by 1,000 miles of Indian territory. Development of the East wing tended to be

---

[4] A survey of MR field leaders in 1990 asked (among other questions) about the extent of importation of foreign ideas and methods, and whether there had been sufficient adaptation to Pakistan's cultures. Responses on this were very mixed, almost equal numbers thinking that there was an appropriate East-West blend, that Western ideas were too prominent, and that more Western contributions were needed (Miles 1993).

hampered by decisions taken far away in the West wing, which itself took many years to settle down after the traumas of Partition and the reception of very large numbers of Muslims leaving India. By the time the East wing fought and gained its independence as Bangladesh, it had rather fallen behind in terms of development, especially for those parts of the population that customarily had very low priority. By the mid 1970s, major cities across the rest of the subcontinent each had at least one organisation and school for mentally retarded children. No such work was reported from Bangladesh, though there were and still are some very backward children casually integrated in ordinary schools (Begum 1991). Finally in 1977 there were meetings in Dhaka among "the parents of the mentally retarded children, psychologists, psychiatrists and social workers who had been deliberating and exchanging views on the problems of mentally retarded children" (SCEMRB Report 1977-81, 1982, 10). These meetings led to the formation of the Society for Care and Education of Mentally Retarded, Bangladesh (SCEMRB) in December 1977, followed shortly afterwards by the opening of a special class for children with MR, in the grounds of an ordinary school.

Later events, in particular a power struggle between parents and professionals, seem to have led to some revision of accounts of this NGO's earliest days. Thus in 1994 the President of SCEMRB asserted that, like the Nordic organisation with which it soon developed a partnership, SCEMRB was always "basically a Parents Organisation", and that although some professionals did get involved, "it basically retains the character of a parents' organization" (Barua, 1994). This view of its origins is contradicted by the First Report of SCEMRB covering 1977-1981, written by one of the founding parents, stating that

> At the time of the formation of the Society when its programmes and projects were adopted, the concept of parents associations and involvement of parents in the activities of the Society was not there. For the first time in our Second National Conference held in June, 1981 Mr Sigurd Gohli Secretary General of the Norwegian Association for the Mentally Retarded defined the concept of parents association and explained how parents could be involved in the various projects and programmes for the welfare of the retarded. Programmes and projects as envisaged in the original scheme of things were to be managed by the professionals under the guidance of the Society. (ibid. p.18)

By 1980, four special education classes had started, the fourth being for Dhaka slum children (SCEMRB Report 1977-81, pp. 18-19). The teachers were a mixture of young psychology graduates and mothers, some of the latter working without salary to start with. Guidance was provided by Dr. Sultana Zaman, a senior psychologist, who played a key role in the early development of SCEMRB, and eventually left to form another NGO with a stronger research and development focus, the Bangladesh Protibondhi Foundation. The SCEMRB early years apparently saw much support from well-wishers and businesses in Dhaka, many donations of goods, time and money, including substantial amounts from the Government. The SCEMRB Report 1977-81 notes under the heading "Affiliated Bodies" that "The Society has affiliated similar Associations set up in Chittagong and Rajshahi." This 'affiliation' soon turned into 'assimilation', as large amounts of Nordic aid began to be channelled through SCEMRB at Dhaka.

It thus appears that the earliest developments were fairly similar to those in Pakistan, though occurring some 15 years later; but change soon took place as a result of partnership with the Nordic NGO, which specialised in MR and which emphasised parent control. Instead of each city developing one or more independent NGOs concerned with MR, which would raise their own funds, run their own service centre and pursue their own goals, the main pattern that emerged in Bangladesh was to have one national NGO based in Dhaka, controlling branches which benefited by substantial foreign aid via Dhaka. The aid partnership began in 1982, and by 1995 branches had extended to 36 towns or rural bases. Special classes and special schools were opened, vocational workshops were tried out, some success was achieved with agro-based rural training projects, and there is some ongoing extension with Government assistance, to provide more formal services. Initially through the aid partnership, and later with extension by the efforts of the Bangladesh Protibondhi Foundation, the country has had access to a wide range of modern information about MR - the accumulated concepts, knowledge, skills and designs of modern Europe in this field. The accelerated development of branches, and large Nordic subsidy to professionals' salaries, has spread know-how to small towns across urban Bangladesh. Without the Nordic organisation's pressure and support, formal services and information would most probably have been confined still to the major cities, with perhaps one or two rural experiments. There are also now formal structures in place for professional training and support, through Nordic-aided training institutions established at or near Dhaka, and Dhaka University's Department of Special Education. Given the vast political, economic, social and cultural differences between Norway and Bangladesh, the absence of historical links between the countries, and the colossal difficulties and natural disasters experienced by Bangladesh throughout this period, the achievement has been substantial.

The sustainability of the whole exercise remains uncertain however, given that Nordic aid could not be expected to continue indefinitely, and in fact has already begun to be cut back. The issue concerns not only the daily services, special classes and professional salaries, but the continued existence of a national advocacy organisation having some access to government planning and finance. The Nordic side of the partnership has tried to emphasise the importance of advocacy, and of the inclusion of mentally retarded people in the ordinary government education, health and welfare services - since this sort of advocacy has been an important factor in the development of well-funded inclusive services benefiting mentally retarded people and their families in Nordic countries. Yet an evaluation team in 1988 noticed that this sort of advocacy was one of the weaker trends in SCEMRB. The stronger trend was towards separate facilities, with each branch aiming to have its own building on its own plot of land, in which it would 'do its own thing' (Hoel et al. 1988, pp. 14, 16). Other subsequent evaluations have noticed the tendency of powerful, urban parents to secure resources for the benefit of their own MR children, ignoring the fact that the great majority of families have had no help at all, not even an information pamphlet or ten minutes of well-informed counselling. The drive to build separate facilities, and the concentration of resources to benefit a few, continue to be prominent in the late 1990s. The Nordic ambition to see integrated, decentralised services has been strongly resisted by parents who joined SCEMRB to secure benefits for their own child and who have not wanted to see those benefits 'diluted' by being shared with hundreds and thousands of other families.[5]

The ability of SCEMRB branch leadership to maintain an independent line, quietly rejecting the central policies of the NGO and its major funder, was one of the features that puzzled an idealistic but increasingly disillusioned Nordic advisor who spent several years with SCEMRB. He reported a curious form of organisational paralysis at the heart of SCEMRB:

> The lack of an effective administration and organisational control, decision- and policy making have led to a situation where the branches feel free to run their business in whatever way they like. And they are doing exactly that. (Haanes 1994)

Nevertheless, this situation could coexist with his apparently contrary complaint a little later, that

> It is, as we all know, a sad fact that the SCEMRB constitution of today creates an undemocratic and highly centralised structure of power and control in the organisation. (Haanes 1995)

The solution to the conundrum of how branches could do whatever they liked, despite the centralisation of power and control, may be found in the fact that, as also in Pakistan, very few NGOs or branches paid any attention to what was written in their constitution. The realities of power and action lay with the personalities in each place, and in the unwritten laws and hidden currents with which they moved.

---

[5] Such an attitude reflects a broader trend in urban Bangladesh, documented strikingly by Blanchet (1996), in which middle-class children are driven forward almost abusively through the 'examination hell' by ambitious families, while many children of the poor are grossly exploited by rapacious employers. Similar trends were reported from the 1970s and 1980s in urban India and Pakistan.

The author's comparative impression of NGO development and MR services is based on a much longer involvement with Pakistani NGOs than with SCEMRB and its branches, so there may be some bias or imbalance here. Nonetheless, the impression is that NGO services in these two countries have reached a broadly similar level of development, though each has strengths that are lacking in the other. So far as concerns the type of services provided, there has also been some convergence over time in the sort of educational policies and issues affecting both countries, e.g. debate over separate or integrated services, rights and inclusion, as outlined by Miles and Hossain (1999).

The Pakistani NGOs have the strengths of diversity, in their goals, approaches and methods, in their local and external fund-raising links, in the varied drives and motivations of the leaders in different places, in the varied mixture of parents, professionals and other concerned people, even in the various sorts of competition between NGOs. They may not make a coherent impression on national planning or on the international scene, but they are well rooted all over urban Pakistan, and are unlikely to disappear. Even if some foreign donors pull out, others would be likely to continue. When new opportunities arise, or innovations appear from abroad, there is sufficient flexibility for one or another NGO to try them out, without the others needing to commit themselves. Even if there is no effective national platform, the government periodically takes soundings among the field leaders in various places. The Bangladeshi national NGO and branches have the strength of unity- SCEMRB is known to government and national media as the body that speaks on MR; its experiences are to some extent cumulative, so that mistakes made and lessons learnt in one branch can be communicated to all; it produces and circulates one or two magazines, rather than thirty competing newsletters; the potential exists, and is occasionally realised, for a strong, well-established branch to assist a small struggling branch. SCEMRB can also credibly represent Bangladesh at international meetings, and perhaps has grown sufficiently confident that it can resist pressure from external donors to adopt western trends that it knows to be culturally inappropriate. It is, however, vulnerable unless it can broaden its financial support base.

The weaknesses of the NGOs in both countries are those common to NGOs worldwide: the lack of managerial competence, poor accounting and administration, narrow vision and weak planning, channelling of resources to the middle classes rather than to those in greater need, dominance of a small number of personalities, party spirit and politicking, and so on.

The Pakistani NGOs have made some efforts to obtain the benefits of a national platform, but any such organisation would probably remain weak because its members are very reluctant to give up any of their independence and competitiveness. In practice, the Bangladeshi organisational branches have been in some ways like the Pakistani NGOs, acting independently of their central core, and some of them contemplate an independent future in case the national organisation fails to sustain itself. Pakistan built up to its present resources over a longer period, and with a stronger economy; on the other hand, Bangladesh started its formal services in time to catch the 'disability development decade' of the 1980s, and the foreign partner put very substantial resources at its disposal. On the evidence available, neither development pattern seems clearly superior to the other.

Planners and aid agencies contemplating assistance to disability organisations would therefore be well advised to take a flexible position and evaluate the merits, arguments and earlier history of the particular country and situation in any proposal. Western disability NGOs in particular should think long and hard before imposing their own preoccupations on countries that may well be at a different stage of development, with different needs and preoccupations. Since the late 1970s, some western organisations have first supported NGOs building special schools in developing countries; then switched their emphasis toward special units attached to ordinary schools. Next some of them decided that NGOs should provide no services but should campaign for government provision of integrated education, while others backed NGOs attempting Community-Based Rehabilitation. More recently, whatever was done had to be led by disabled people's groups, with special focus on women's rights; and now what is considered to be really needed is 'Inclusion', involving a total reconceptualisation of what education (or the whole of life) is all about. To implement any one of these policy changes with the slightest chance of effectiveness probably required from 20 to 50 years, as well as strong political, parental and professional motivation - none of which has been present. The good intentions behind these policies shifts is not in question - but for aid to be enabling rather than disabling, it should respect the realities as perceived by the recipient, rather than the ideological viewpoint of the donor.

REFERENCES

Barua, D. P. (1994): SCEMRB: a brief profile. In: *Souvenir Brochure of SCEMRB* distributed at 12th Asian Conference on Mental Retardation, Colombo, September 1995, pp. 11-12.

Begum, K. (1991): Identifying learning difficulties and adoption of remedial measures for primary school children, Teacher's World. *Journal of Education and Research* 14 (2) 1-7.

Bhandara, M. P. (1971): *Cyclostyled letter Ref. No. SDC/1002/71 dated 20th March 1971*, headed: School for Disabled Children -Funds for, from Mr. M.P. Bhandara, President, Managing Committee, Chambeeli School, D-103, Satellite Town, Rawalpindi.

Blanchet, T. (1996): *Lost Innocence, Stolen Childhoods*. Dhaka: University Press.

Danielou, A. with Gopala Iyer, T. V. (transl.) (1993): *Manimekhalai (The Dancer with the Magic Bowl) by Merchant-Prince Shattan.* New Delhi: Penguin.

Haanes, K. J. (1994, 1995): *Progress Reports on SCEMRB.* Unpublished.

Haynes, D. E. (1987): From tribute to philanthropy: the politics of gift giving in a Western Indian city, *Journal of Asian Studies* 46: 339-360.

Hoel, V. & Mathias, M. & Rahman, A. (1988): *Consultancy report on SCEMRB* prepared for NORAD, Oslo. Unpublished.

Khan, M. Ahmad (1972): *Social Welfare Services in North-West Frontier Province.* Peshawar: Board of Economic Enquiry NWFP, University of Peshawar.

Kozlowski, G. C. (1995): Imperial authority, benefactions and endowments (awq]f) in Mughal India, *Journal of the Economic and Social History of the Orient* 38: 355-370.

The Mahabharata, transl. K. M. Ganguli (1883-1896), reprint 1993, from 1970 edition, New Delhi: Munshiram Manoharlal.

Makhdum, S. A. (1961): *Special Education in West Pakistan.* Lahore: West Pakistan Bureau of Education.

Miles, M. (1993): Mental handicap services: practical trends in Pakistan, *European Journal of Special Needs Education* 8: 45-58.

Miles, M. (1998a): Development of Community Based Rehabilitation in Pakistan: bringing mental handicap into focus, *International Journal of Development, Disability & Education* 45: 431-448.

Miles, M. (1998b): Professional and family responses to mental retardation in East Bengal and Bangladesh, 1770s-1990s, *International Journal of Educational Development* 18: 487-499.

Miles, M. (1999): *Some historical responses to disability in South Asia and reflections on service provision.* Unpublished Ph.D. thesis, University of Birmingham, UK.

Miles, M. & Hossain, F. (1999): Rights and disabilities in educational provision in Pakistan and Bangladesh: roots, rhetoric, reality, in: F. Armstrong & L. Barton (eds): *Disability, Human Rights, and Education: cross cultural perspectives,* 67-86, Buckingham: Open UP.

Muslim, A. S. (1993): *Mental Retardation in Pakistan.* Karachi: Society for Children in Need of Special Attention.

Pakistan Society for the Welfare of Mentally Retarded Children (1993): *Introductory Brochure.* Lahore.

Peters, H. & Rehman, F. (1988): *Community Directed Rehabilitation for Disabled Children in NWFP Pakistan.* Peshawar: Frontier Association for the Mentally Handicapped.

Rashid, S. K. (1978): *Wakf Administration in India, a socio-legal study.* New Delhi: Vikas.

SCEMRB Report 1977-81. Dhaka: Society for Care and Education of Mentally Retarded Bangladesh.

Sanyal, R. (1977): Indian participation in organized charity in early Calcutta, 1818-1866, *Bengal Past and Present* 96: 97-113.

Sherring, M. A. (1875): *Hand-Book for Visitors to Benares*. Calcutta: Newman.

Stillman, N. A. (1975): Charity and social services in Medieval Islam, *Societas: a review of social history* 5 (2) 105-115.

Strickland, C. F. (1939): Chapters on `Co-operation' and on `Voluntary effort and social welfare', in: E. Blunt (ed.) *Social Service in India*. 312-343, 372-398, Ldn: HMSO.

14. NON-GOVERNMENTAL ORGANISATIONS IN BANGLADESH: AN ASSESSMENT OF THEIR LEGAL STATUS

Mokbul Morshed Ahmad

INTRODUCTION

The paper will first outline the overall situation of Non-Government Organisations in Bangladesh, then set out the legal issues in detail and finally make proposals for improvements. State-NGO relations in Bangladesh have moved through stages of indifference and ambivalence (News from Bangladesh 1999e; Lewis and Sobhan 1999; White 1999; Khan 1999; compare Baig 1999 on Pakistan; Sen 1999 on India). In other parts of the Muslim world, state has in general been sceptical or strict towards NGOs, human rights and community groups (Huband *et al.* 1999; Huband 1999; Galpin 1999). When the state in Bangladesh tried to control the activities of NGOs, the donors put pressure on the state, which responded by imposing more paperwork on the NGOs, thus increasing their transaction costs. The state has failed to make NGOs more transparent, functionally or financially. So, NGOs can easily violate laws because of the weakness of the state and their own strength which over time has been fed by the donors.

NGOS IN BANGLADESH

Since the independence of Bangladesh in 1971, the state has largely failed to assist the poor or reduce poverty, and NGOs have grown dramatically, ostensibly to fill this gap. There are more and bigger NGOs in Bangladesh than in any other country of equivalent size. The Association of Development Agencies in Bangladesh (ADAB) had a total membership of 886 NGOs in December 1997, of which 231 were central and 655 chapter (local) members (ADAB, 1998), the ADAB Directory lists 1007 NGOs including 376 non-member NGOs. The NGO Affairs Bureau of the Government of Bangladesh (GOB), which has to approve all foreign grants to NGOs working in Bangladesh, released grants worth about 250 million US $ in FY 1996-97 to 1,132 NGOs, of which 997 are local and 135 are foreign (NGO Affairs Bureau 1998). NGOs have mainly functioned in order to service the needs of the landless, usually with foreign donor funding as a counter-point to the state's efforts (Lewis 1993).

Despite their numbers, NGOs have brought little change in levels of poverty. Even the largest NGOs in Bangladesh taken together cover only a fraction of the population: perhaps only 10-20 percent of landless households (Hashemi 1995). NGOs in Bangladesh have not originated from Grass Root Organisations (GROs) in civil society. Rather it is NGO workers who set up groups, which clients then join to get microcredit and other services. Most Bangladeshi NGOs are totally dependent upon foreign funds. The volume of foreign funds to NGOs in Bangladesh has been increasing over the years and stood at just under 18 percent of all foreign 'aid' to the country in FY 1995-96. Donors increased their funding from 464 NGO projects in 1990-91 to 746 in 1996-97, a 60 per cent increase in six years; the total amount disbursed showed a 143 per cent increase over the period (NGO Affairs Bureau 1998). However, the disbursement of funds to NGOs is highly skewed. The top 15 NGOs accounted for 84 per cent of all allocation to NGOs in 1991-92, and 70 percent in 1992-93 (Hashemi 1995). NGO dependence on donor grants has kept the whole operation highly subsidised. For example, the annual working costs of BRAC's (one of the largest NGOs in Bangladesh) branch-level units are still more than three times their locally generated income (Montgomery et al. 1996).

NGOs in Bangladesh have shifted their focus from social mobilisation in the 1970s and 80s to economic changes for their clients in the 1990s (Hashemi 1995). This change in focus has happened for several main reasons. *Firstly*, NGOs' struggle on issues like access to *khas* (state) land put them in conflict with both the state and the local elite. NGOs role in the anti autocracy movement was fostered by major political parties (1990). In 1996, NGOs took part in a successful movement for elections which antagonised the government in power at the same time. *Secondly*, NGOs are trying to become self-reliant through involvement in business or microcredit operations. Nowadays, very few NGOs are engaged in social movements, which marks a division in the NGO community. Not a single NGO in Bangladesh talk against corruption which is a major social problem in Bangladesh.

Table 1. Stages of changes in the activities of NGOs.

Date	Political System	Activities
1971-1990	Military, quasi-military rule	Relief, social mobilisation, anti-autocracy movement
1991-	Democracy	Relief only after natural hazards, business, microcredit, limited social movements by some (against fundamentalists, for sex workers, women)

LEGAL STATUS OF NGOS, PAST AND PRESENT

The term 'legal status of NGOs' means law as it pertains to NGOs[1]. Most of the ordinances and regulations promulgated by the state were aimed at controlling the receipt of foreign money by NGOs or activities. The most significant steps of Ershad Government regarding NGOs were the abolition of the NGO Standing Committee, the creation of the NGO Affairs Bureau (NAB) and the appointment of an Advisor for NGO Affairs with Ministerial status (White 1999). The NAB started functioning with effect from 1st March, 1990. It was headed by a Director-General and began as the contact point between the State and various foreign and local NGOs receiving foreign donations. As all NGO activities came under the purview of the 'President's Secretariat Public Division', NGOs were supposed to be regulated by the NAB instead of the Department of Social Welfare. Within a short period of time, the Bureau had shown promise by its quick clearance of NGO applications. However, the procedures still remained complex, and needed further improvement.

THE LAW AND NGOS IN BANGLADESH

The state in Bangladesh requires each NGO to register formally with NAB, and to renew this registration every five years. Each project must be approved in advance by the NAB, as must all foreign funding. Each NGO must receive all funding through a single, specific bank account, and the bank must submit full reports to the central bank, which then reports to the NAB and to the Economic Relations Division (ERD) of the Ministry of Finance. The NAB also regulates the use of foreign consultants. For projects and programmes of disaster-relief, requirements are similar but the NAB must decide more rapidly. Each NGO must submit annual auditor's reports to the NAB, having appointed its auditors from the list approved by the NAB. Penalties for false statements, failures to submit declarations or other contraventions of the law include heavy fines payable by the NGO and/or imprisonment of NGO directors. The transaction costs for NGOs in securing permissions and approvals are very high, in both avoidable delays and unnecessary paperwork. Far too much unnecessary information is required, usually in multiple copies.

State regulations define the term 'Voluntary Activity' as an activity undertaken, with partial or complete support from external sources, by any person or organisation to render voluntary services pertaining to agricultural, relief, missionary, educational, cultural, vocational, social welfare and other developmental activities in the country. Although the definition seems to cover almost all kinds of voluntary activities, the state retains the right to include or exclude any activity as "voluntary"[2]. The state apparently intended to widen the scope of the definition in order to prevent both the donors and recipients from making or receiving grants/donations in contravention of official ordinances[3].

The ordinances/regulations/circulars vested the NAB all its responsibilities regarding co-ordination, regulation and monitoring of foreign and foreign assisted non-government voluntary organisations and individuals working in Bangladesh. The NAB is charged with certain responsibilities[4]. While considering the application for registration, the NAB is required to seek approval from the Home Ministry[5].

Projects may be for one or multiple years. NGOs can submit a five year project proposal, commensurate with an identified priority area of the five year plan of the state. The NAB arranges approval and release of the funds on a priority basis for such projects. The targets specified in the project proposal, however, must be achieved within the stipulated period. Usually funds for the following year can be released for the project if its implementation strategy and achievement of target for the year is considered to be satisfactory by the Bureau (Circular: Section 7 (h) 1993).

Existing NGO regulations make exception for projects for assistance to disaster-affected areas. For disaster rehabilitation programmes, NGOs have to submit their project proposal with requisite details on a prescribed proforma FD-6 (Circular: 7.1(a) 1993). The NAB communicates its decisions with 21 days from the day of the receipt of the project proposal and forwards it to the relevant Ministry for its opinion. The Ministry must send its decision to the NAB within 14 days (Circular: Section 7.1(b) 1993).

The state and its machinaries have from time to time introduced several rules and procedures but, due to their complexity and weakness of the state, NGOs can easily evade them. The rules for receipt and use of foreign donations[6] and the banking transactions of NGOs[7] are interesting examples. These are elaborated below:

SUBMISSION OF ANNUAL REPORTS

NGOs are required to prepare annual reports on their activities within three months of the end of the financial year and send copies to the NAB, ERD, the relevant Ministry, Divisional Commissioner(s), Deputy Commissioners and the Bangladesh Bank.

POWER OF INSPECTION

The State may, at any time inspect the accounts and other documents of NGOs. The state may require the NGO to submit a declaration as notified in the official gazette (Ordinance No. XLVI: Section 4(1) 1978). Failure to produce any accounts or other documents or failure to furnish any statement or information by the NGO is a contravention of state regulations (Ordinance XLVI: Section 4(3) 1978). The NAB has the responsibility and power to audit and inspect the accounts of NGOs (Circular: Section 10(a) 1993).

The accounts of any NGO must be audited by the person/s appointed by the relevant NGO or persons enlisted/approved by the NAB. Audit reports must be submitted to the NAB within two months of the end of the financial year.

From the above discussion we have a clear picture of the manner/procedure regarding the way the state of Bangladesh regulates those NGOs which finance charitable work through foreign donations. The donor agencies led by The World Bank (WB) have strongly supported the formulation of the State's policy on NGOs, particularly in the direction of streamlining the administrative and legal framework within which NGOs operate, to increase their effectiveness (Zareen 1996).

CRITICAL ASSESSMENT

NGOs in Bangladesh have increasingly become subject to question and criticism from state, political parties, intellectuals and the public in general. Let us critically discuss the issues in brief from a legal standpoint.

Recently there has been allegations of misuse of funds, gender discrimination, nepotism against a large NGO called Gono Sahajja Sangstha (GSS). A state and another donor investigation found that the rural level female workers of GSS were compelled to go on maternity leave without pay. They also found that GSS bought lands worth millions of Taka to build its headquarters in Dhaka. The donors stopped funding the NGO too (Kabir 1999; News from Bangladesh 1999c). In the long process of NGO development in Bangladesh, many NGOs have certainly empowered themselves with structures and buildings, while empowerment of the poor beyond better services has been rather limited. Recently, NGO activities and expenditures came under fire in the National Parliament and other forums (The Daily Star 1999b; NFB 1999d). One Member of Parliament (MP) alleged that some NGOs raised money on false promises of jobs and credit, but misappropriated it. Another MP claimed that some NGOs make loans at the high rate of 14% and resort to "inhuman torture" on debtors who fail to repay on time (News from Bangladesh 1999a). The relevant minister gave a face-saving answer to all these allegations but in reality there is poor control by the state on NGOs in Bangladesh. This was reiterated by the head of NAB in another occasion (News from Bangladesh 1999b).

Any powerful NGO may deliberately manipulate the Ministry of Home Affairs or the relevant Ministry when it has not delivered an opinion within the stipulated time (as mentioned in Circular 1993) so that the application may be passed without any objection. If this happens, the illegal issue would not be eliminated.

According to law[8], no person or organisation may receive or spend foreign loans/grants without the prior state approval. The NAB Report submitted to the Prime Minister's Secretariat in 1992 stated that various NGOs had disbursed Taka 1.5 billion without prior state permission in the financial year 1990 to 1991. Quite often, large amounts of money come into the country illegally. 'The Salvation Army' received Taka 12.5 million without the state approval (Government Report 1992); similarly, 'Sheba Shongho' spent Taka 13.5 million without state approval, and the 'Finnish Free Mission' also violated state instructions (Report-1, 18th August, 1992; *Bhorer Kagoj* 1992).

According to a Government Inspection Report (1992), senior officials of some NGOs quite often travel abroad and, without state approval, obtain foreign donations. According to this report the accounts provided by the NGOs may fail to match those provided by the Bangladesh Bank, although according to law[9], if any organisation wants to carry out a charitable programme, then it should receive any foreign currency through an approved bank in Bangladesh. This restriction was imposed to give the state a true picture of the total amount of foreign currency in the hands of NGOs, as well as giving it indirect control of the flow of foreign funds to the NGO sector. Yet, according to another act[10], any organisation/person can bring any amount of foreign currency into Bangladesh. Therefore, as a result of this dual system, no-one can know the total amount of foreign currency actually received by any NGO. Close observation of NGO activities in Bangladesh would further substantiate the problem.

According to a nineteenth century Act[11], voluntary societies cannot undertake business oriented projects. As in the same Act, upon the dissolution of the society and payment of all its debts and liabilities, no property whatsoever shall be paid to or distributed among the members of the society but should be vested in the managing committee. In a 1961 Ordinance there is provision for gaining profit in order to create job opportunities. Both the Act and Ordinance apply to the same cases. As a consequence, some NGOs are flourishing simultaneously as service-oriented organisations and as profit-oriented business organisations. The state is also being deprived of tax by NGOs taking advantage of loopholes in the regulations. Some senior officials of certain NGOs have used loopholes to become affluent[12].

BRAC is currently alleged to be running successful businesses like a commercial organisation, contrary to its charitable status. BRAC's cold storage, press, a marketing organisation named 'Aarong', a real estate company, and a restaurant etc. are highly profitable. Recently BRAC has received state approval to open a commercial bank for micro lending (The Financial Times 1998). BRAC is also said to be planning to open a private university. BRAC provides no accounts of their commercial organisation's income or expenditure to any state department. White (1999) points out that BRAC generates 31 per cent of its income from its business sources. As BRAC is not registered under the Ordinance of 1961, if ever the dissolution of BRAC occurs then all its property will be vested in the managing committee. BRAC possesses more than 50 modern automobiles (Zarren 1996).

The Government Report (1992) reports a complaint against PROSHIKA (another large NGO) that, although PROSHIKA is registered under 1961 Ordinance, it has still developed a transport company of 28 buses at a cost of 30 million Taka. At a cost of 15 million Taka, PROSHIKA has also established a press and a garment industry and is investing Taka 5 million in a video library. Recently it has started an internet and software business. In some cases, service-oriented NGO projects are basically market-oriented, with the objective of earning profits through long term capital investment. BRAC's cold storage project (costing Taka seventy million) and Savar Ganosastha Kendro's (GK, another large NGO) highly profitable clinic, university and medicine businesses are striking examples. Allegations have also been made against GSS, another large NGO which used donors' funds to open printing press, media business but not audited and taxed as per rules of the state (Kabir 1999). The Finance minister told in a seminar that most NGOs are engaged in banking violating the law (The Independent 1999).

The Government Report (1992) states that Association of Development Agencies in Bangladesh -- ADAB's dishonesty is evident as it has several bank accounts. This violates state rules, when any NGO must receive foreign donations through a single bank account (Regulation Rules: Section 4(4) 1978). The power to appoint any state-registered firm as an auditor is currently vested in the NGOs themselves, which is alleged to have resulted in auditors giving favourable reports on their clients. The NAB is further reported to have 2 audit supervisors but not a single auditor, so that the state is unable to obtain a clear picture of the actual status of NGOs in the country. Only a random sample of audit reports are examined, so most NGOs are not reviewed.

After audit and inspection, if a complaint is lodged against an NGO, virtually no appropriate action is taken. Usually a note is passed to the NGO to correct the error, which is a trivial measure. Due to the strong support of donors for NGOs, the state has in the recent past had to scrap its own desire to withdraw the registration of a number of NGOs and even to change the head of the NAB, who had appeared tough with NGOs which had indulged in irregularities (Hashemi 1995). When the NAB cancelled the registration of three NGOs for financial irregularities, the head of a diplomatic mission in Dhaka personally intervened, brought the issue to the attention of the Prime Minister's office and got the cancellation order withdrawn. This action created great dissatisfaction among the officials of the Bureau (Hashemi 1995).

NGOs are non-democratic institutions, often dominated or dictated to by one individual, and many have a serious ownership problem. As NGOs are heavily dependent on foreign resources, then, in the absence of accountability, the flow of money from the outside can make the NGOs corrupt, controversial and autocratic (Zarren 1996). Despite the negative effects, ironically real in most cases, NGOs are accountable to the donor countries rather than the state of Bangladesh (The Independent, June 14, 1995).

In reality, the State is unable to control the NGOs. The NGOs often work against the directions and decisions of the state. Weak administration on the one hand and strong national and international backing on the other encourage some NGOs to defy the state and to work according to their own whims. In the recent past, the registration of Association of Development Agencies in Bangladesh (ADAB) was cancelled by the NAB but reinstated within a few hours. This was naturally achieved by a powerful international lobby. There is a tug of war between the NAB and the Social Welfare Directorate which gives the NGOs opportunities to break the rules (*The Daily Inquilab*, September 23, 1992; *The Daily Sangbad*, January 6, 1993).

RECOMMENDATIONS

The following recommendations would improve the existing legal status of NGOs in Bangladesh, by reducing bureaucracy, removing legal contradictions and making the NGOs more accountable. Sadly, donors might resent such improvements.

State Rules/Acts/ Ordinances should be replaced/modified to reflect the current critical atmosphere[13]. The state should remove all administrative and procedural bottlenecks created through promulgation of various Ordinances and streamline the existing working procedures, enabling NGOs to complete all formalities within the shortest possible time. The state should appraise the strength and weakness of the measures for regulating the NGOs and ensure promulgation of flexible and effective rules and regulations.

Improving NGO Efficiency

Just to renew an NGO's registration, it takes more than two months to prepare papers which are in the event not thoroughly scrutinised. As the state has the authority, in any case of serious allegations, to cancel the registration of any NGO or stop its activities and inform the donor, then once any NGO is registered, renewal procedures should be simplified.

Some of the Foreign Donation (FD) forms and procedures followed by the NAB are complex and cumbersome. The application forms and procedures should be simplified, through discussion between the GOB and NGOs. With regard to registration, the Home Ministry should give approval/disapproval within sixty days of receiving the application from the NAB regarding the appointment/extension of the tenure of expatriates, within 25 days. Reminders could be sent to the National Security Intelligence (NSI) by the NAB.

Appropriate action should be taken by the administrative Ministries / Divisions / Departments to give their advice to the NAB within 21 days with regard to approval of NGO projects.

To enable NGOs to prepare budgets and implement projects within the time limit of financial year, if the report about a particular NGO is satisfactory, then the NGO could be given clearance for other projects in the same year without further investigation by the NAB.

The existing procedure each year of requiring that projects and clearance of funds be approved by the state should be changed. NGOs which have approval for a project should be able to use foreign funds until the project is completed, with no annual renewal. Since the funds must be received through specific NGO bank accounts, the state will be able to monitor the flow of foreign funds to the NGO sector and to each NGO. It will be the business of NAB officials to check whether an NGO has several bank accounts.

The National Security Intelligence (NSI) should be aware of each NGO's activities so that it is ready to comment on an application without further inquiry. If the NGO had done anything highly objectionable during the last 29 years, it should have been closed and the relevant donor informed.

For NAB approval of projects, the NGOs should be required to submit the names of the members of the Board / Executive Committee and the number of staff positions in each category, not staff names.

Improving The Law

According to a circular[14] , 'No such project would be approved if it offends the feelings of the people of any religion, has adverse effects on the culture and values of the country or if the project is based on a political programme'. Around 90% of the laws in Bangladesh are secular. Around 87% of the population is Muslim (BBS 1998) and Islam is the state religion in Bangladesh. So, there are legal problems in Bangladesh arising from unresolved conflicts in the law. Now, women's independence / women's empowerment programmes are against the beliefs of many strict Muslims, but 'gender-development' is a leading concern of western donors. So, a specific political party could firmly resist women's development and the NGOs would have to end women's development programmes (Chazan 1998). This would be unethical as well as undesirable.

Recently unrest started when Islamic teachers and students organised a general strike in a north-eastern town of Bangladesh and demonstrators attacked a rally of women clients of NGOs and set fire to the offices of several NGOs. Several more were injured. A rally was organised by NGOs which have lent money to millions of poor Bangladeshi women to start small shops or businesses such as poultry breeding and weaving. Several thousand women who benefited from such loans took part. Islamic groups said they objected to women taking part in celebrations to commemorate the 1971 victory over Pakistan which led to the independence of Bangladesh. But NGOs said the fundamentalists had objected to Muslim women going out to work. Human rights groups urged the state to take action against Islamic fundamentalists who attacked women taking part in a rally to commemorate the country's independence struggle (Chazan 1998). Another similar conflict erupted in Faridpur, a district town in central Bangladesh (The Daily Star 1999a). Therefore, the state must clearly define what kinds of programme would affect native culture or strike the sentiment of the people of any religion.

There is supposed to be investigation[15] as to whether any NGO is involved in any political or anti-cultural activity under the guise of a development programme. Now, CARITAS is involved in consciousness-raising, making people aware of their rights, teaching them to be independent, and morally strong and thus empowering people at the grass-roots level. This is not a crime; few people see empowering people as an anti-state activity. This section of the circular should therefore be modified.

Holding NGOs Accountable

The state audit system is ineffective. A mechanism must be developed under which the state officials involved in the development process make regular field visits to NGO programmes. Such state officials should also conduct impact evaluations on completion of the projects, to enhance their insights into the programme dynamics and the operation of NGOs.

Commercial activities of NGOs should be duly taxed and profits from them should be used for development work. The law should be changed accordingly and NAB should make it sure that it is implemented properly. In conformity with law, immediate legal action ought to be taken against the officials of several NGOs who are involved in misappropriation, embezzlement or accused of misconduct, irregularity or law-breaking.

Theoretically, the state is accountable for its activities and programmes to Parliament and ultimately to the public but the NGOs remain unaccountable. This cannot be accepted. NGOs must be regulated by Parliament. If the government can remain above narrow party interests and if the opposition party can remain strong and responsible, then an effective parliamentary committee could be created to scrutinise and evaluate the activities and programmes of the NGOs.

CONCLUSION

In Bangladesh NGOs play a pivotal and pragmatic role when the state does not reach the poor and meet their needs. The NGOs' umbrella body (which is required to elect its executive committee) is not broad-based. Its membership is often confined to friends and relatives and elections to the executive committee are often not properly held. This surely frustrates the potential of NGOs as democratic voluntary organisations. Nevertheless, NGOs cannot function in isolation from the main streams of political, economic and social life in the country. They must conform to certain standards, adhere to state regulations and have their work co-ordinated at state level. NGOs can only complement the state's activity. Due to donor pressure the state cannot ask NGOs to become more transparent and accountable or to co-operate more with the state. The state is very weak in Bangladesh (Wood 1997). Instead the state creates undue hindrances which only increases the transaction costs of NGOs without encouraging or forcing the NGOs to respond more to the needs of the poor.

REFERENCES

ADAB (1998): *Directory of PVDOs/NGDOs in Bangladesh (Ready Reference)*. Dhaka: ADAB.

Baig, Q. (1999): NGO Governing Bodies and Beyond: A Southern Perspective on Third Sector Governance Issues. In Lewis, D. (ed.). *International Perspectives on Voluntary Action Reshaping The Third Sector*. London: Earthscan.

BBS (1998): *Statistical Pocketbook of Bangladesh*. Dhaka: Bangladesh Bureau of Statistics.

Bhorer Kagoj (1992): October 29, 1992 (Daily Newspaper in Bangla).

Chazan, D. (1998): "Aid Offices Set on Fire in Bangladesh". *The Financial Times*. December 9, 1998.

The Daily Star (1999a): "Tension Prevails at Faridpur Over ADAB Conference". *The Daily Star. (Daily News Paper)*. March 6, 1999. (From world wide web).

The Daily Star (1999b): "Kibria on Microfinance Institutions: Time Has come for Regulating Their Lending Activities". *The Daily Star. (Daily News Paper)*. May 7, 1999. (From world wide web).

The Daily Sangbad (1993): January, 6, 1993 (Daily Newspaper in Bangla).

Ebdon, R. (1995): "NGO Expansion and The Fight to Reach The Poor: Gender Implications of NGO Scaling-up in Bangladesh". *IDS Bulletin*. Vol. 26. No. 3. pp. 49-55.

Financial Times (1998): "Bangladesh to Get New Bank for Small Loans". 11th December.

Galpin, R. (1999): "Pakistan Tightens Screw on opposition". *The Guardian*. May, 15, 1999.

Huband, et al. (1999): "Middle Eastern NGOs Strain at The Bonds of Authoritarian Government". *Financial Times*. June 10, 1999.

Huband, M. (1999): "Top Egypt Academics Repudiate Draft Law". *Financial Times*. May 25, 1999.

Hashemi, S. M. (1995): NGO Accountability in Bangladesh: Beneficiaries, Donors and State. In: Edwards, M. & Hulme, D. (eds.) *Non-governmental Organisations - Performance and Accountability Beyond the Magic Bullet*. London: Earthscan Publications.

The Independent (1999): "Most NGOs are Engaged in Banking Violating Law:

Kibria". August, 17 (from World wide web).

The Daily Inquilab (1992): September 23, 1992 (News Paper in Bangla).

Islam, M. A. (1995): Editorial. *The Independent.* (Daily News Paper).

Kabir, N. (1999): "In a Mess: One of The Better-known NGOs Faces Charges of Irregularities". *The Daily Star,* May, 25. (from World wide web).

Khan, T. (1999): "Government Orders Action Against NGOs, Human Rights Groups". *The Independent.* August, 3. (from World wide web).

Lewis, D. & Sobhan, B. (1999): "Routes of Funding, Roots of Trust? Northern NGOs, Southern NGOs, Donors and The Rise of Direct Funding". *Development and Change.* Vol. 9. Nos. 1 &2. pp. 117-129.

Lewis, D. J. (1993): NGO-Government Interaction in Bangladesh. In: Farrington, J. & Lewis, D. J. (eds.) *Non-Governmental Organisations and The State in Asia Rethinking Roles in Sustainable Agricultural Development.* London: Routledge.

Montgomery, R. et al. (1996): Credit for The Poor in Bangladesh - The BRAC Rural Development Programme and The Government Thana Resource Development and Employment Programme. In: Hulme, D. & Mosley, P. (eds.) (1996): *Finance Against Poverty.* Vol. 2. London: Routledge.

News from Bangladesh (1999a): "NGO Activities Come Under Fire in JS". *NFB (The Daily Interactive Edition).* February 5, 1999 (From world wide web).

News from Bangladesh (1999b): "Government Won't Control NGO Activities, Says DG". *NFB (The Daily Interactive Edition).* March 3, 1999 (From world wide web).

News from Bangladesh (1999c): "Donors Block Tk. 1.5b Fund for GSS". *NFB (The Daily Interactive Edition).* May 7, 1999 (From world wide web).

News from Bangladesh (1999d): "PKSF's Call to Hold NGOs in Leash". *NFB (The Daily Interactive Edition).* May 10, 1999 (From world wide web).

News from Bangladesh (1999e): "Restrictions on NGO Activities Likely". *NFB (The Daily Interactive Edition).* October 8, 1999 (From world wide web).

NGO Affairs Bureau (1998): *Flow of Foreign Grant Fund Through NGO Affairs Bureau at a Glance.* Dhaka: NGO Affairs Bureau, PM's Office/GOB.

Report of the NAB for the Prime Minister (1992): "There are several complaints of irregularity and corruption against the NGOs", *Bhorer Kagoj.* 29 July, 1992 (Daily Newspaper in Bangla).

Reza, H. (1992): "Main report, NGO: New Challenge for the State and Government", *Kagoj.* 31 August, 1992 (Weekly Magazine in Bangla).

Salamon, L. M. & Anheier, H. K. (1997): Toward a Common Definition. In: Salamon, L. M. & Anheier, H. K. (eds.): *Defining The Nonprofit Sector A Cross-national Analysis.* Manchester: Manchester University Press.

Sen, S. (1999): "Some Aspects of State-NGO Relations in India in The Post-Independence Era". *Development and Change.* Vol. 30. pp. 327-355.

Task-Force Report (1992): *Report of the Task-Forces on Bangladesh Development Strategies for the 1990s : Managing the Development Process.* Vol. 1 & 2, Dhaka: University Press Limited.

White, S. (1999): "NGOs, Civil Society, and The State in Bangladesh: The Politics of Representing The Poor". *Development and Change.* Vol. 30. pp. 307-326.

Wood, G. D. (1997): States Without Citizens: The Problem of The Franchise State. In: Edwards, M. & Hulme, D. (eds.): *NGOs, States and Donors - Too Close for Comfort?* London: Macmillan.

World Bank (1996): *The World Bank's Partnership with Nongovernmental Organisations.* Washington D. C: Participation and NGO Group, Poverty and Social Policy Department / The World Bank

Zarren, F. (1996): "The Legal Status of NGOs in Bangladesh: A Critical Assessment". *Social Science Review.* Vol. XIII. No. 2. pp. 67-90.

List of Government Ordinances/Rules/Working Procedures :

(i) The Foreign Donations (Voluntary Activities) Regulation Ordinance 1978 : Ordinance No. XLVI of 1978.

(ii) The Foreign Donations (Voluntary Activities) Regulation Rules, 1978 : No. S.R.O. 329-l/78.

(iii) The Foreign Contributions (Regulation) Ordinance, 1982. Ordinance No. XXXI of 1982.

(iv) Working Procedure of Foreign assisted Bangladeshi Non-Government Voluntary Organization (NGOs) A Circular : 22.43.3.1.0.46.93-478, dt. 27-07-1993.

From a daily Newspaper in English; The Independent :

(i) The NGO experience : positive and negative aspects, Julid Rosette ; 6-12-1995.

(ii) Grass-root level intervention : Meghna Guhathakurta : 30-1-1996.

(iii) Keeping up with the pace of development : NGO's role : Md. Monowar Hossain : 29-1-1996.

[1] In 1860, the then Provincial Government of Bengal promulgated the Societies Registration Act No. XXI to improve the legal position of societies for the promotion of literature, science or the fine arts, for diffusion of knowledge or for charitable purposes. The First Ordinance No XLVI of 1961 was promulgated on 2nd December, 1961 by the Martial Law Administration of President Ayub Khan. It made registration mandatory for all NGOs working in what was then East Pakistan and made the Director of Social Welfare responsible for ensuring registration. The Foreign Donations (Voluntary Activities) Regulation Ordinance 1978 was promulgated on 15th November 1978 by President Ziaur Rahman to regulate the receipts and expenditure of foreign donations for voluntary activities. The Foreign Donations (Voluntary Activities) Regulation Rules were promulgated on 12th December, 1978 requiring all NGOs intending to receive foreign funds to be registered under specified prescribed rules. The (Army General) Ershad Government promulgated the Foreign Contributions (Regulations) Ordinance 1982 on 6th September, which reiterated that no individual representing NGOs or the organisations themselves would be allowed to give or receive any foreign contribution without prior permission from the state. The government amended the Foreign Donations (Voluntary Activities) Regulation Rules 1978 on 14th May, 1990.

[2] The Foreign Donations (Voluntary Activities) Regulation Ordinance, 1978 (hereafter FDRO, 1978), for example, defined 'foreign donations' as donations, contributions or grants of any kind made for any voluntary activity in Bangladesh by any foreign government or organisation or a citizen of a foreign state, or by any Bangladeshi citizen living or working abroad (Ordinance XLVI : 1978). The foreign contributions (Regulation/Ordinance, 1982), hereafter FCO, 1982, replaced the term itself by 'foreign contribution', defined as any donation, grant or assistance made by any government, organisation or citizen of a foreign state (Ordinance XXXI : Section 3 : 1982). According to FCO, 1982, any foreign payment, in cash or kind, even a ticket for a journey abroad, has to be considered as a foreign contribution.

[3] The ordinances and regulations are:

a) The Foreign Donations (Voluntary Activities) Regulation Ordinances, 1978.
b) The Foreign Donations (Voluntary Activities) Regulation Rules, 1979.
c) The Foreign Contributions (Regulation) Ordinance, 1982.
d) Working procedure for Foreign and Foreign assisted Bangladeshi Non-Government Voluntary Organizations, 1993.

[4] The Responsibilities are:
a) Arranging 'one-stop service' for NGO registration and processing of project proposal, NGOs are not required to go to any other office or authority for this purposes. (Circular : Section 2: 1993).
b) Approving project proposals submitted by NGOs, release project funds approve appointments of expatriate officials/consultants and their tenure of services (Circular: Section 2: 1993).

c) Scrutinizing and evaluating reports and statements submitted by NGOs.

d) Coordinating, monitoring, inspecting and evaluating NGO programmes and auditing their income and expenditure of accounts.

e) Collecting fees/charges fixed by the government.

f) Examining and taking necessary action on the basis of reports on NGO programmes.

g) Enlisting Chartered Accounts for auditing NGO accounts.

h) Approving receipts of 'one-time contribution' by NGOs. Such contribution is made for buying equipment or for construction of a house/building (Circular :Section 2: 1993).

NAB is also responsible for maintaining communication with concerned Ministries / Agencies on subjects related to operations of NGOs in the country and for obtaining views / opinions from these agencies when required. Government ordinance / regulations requires necessary assistance and co-operation from concerned Ministries / Divisions, other Subordinate Departments / Directories, Divisional Commissioners and Deputy Commissioners for smooth discharge of the stipulated responsibilities of NAB. The Ordinances / Regulations also require that different Ministries / Divisions of the government and their subordinate offices will consult NAB prior to entering any Agreement / Memorandum of Understanding (MOU) with foreign and foreign assisted Bangladeshi NGOs. Before signing such Agreements / MOUs the concerned NGO shall have to be registered under section 3(2) of the Foreign Donations (Voluntary Activities) Regulation Ordinance 1978 (Circular : Section 4: 1993). Such agreements (MOU) are usually signed between an NGO and the government for programmes like running a certain number of schools on behalf of the government, or collaborative programmes like Expanded Immunization Programme.

[5] The Home Ministry is required to give its decision within 60 days of receipt of the letter from the NAB. In considering the application, the Home Ministry is expected to look into the following matters:

(a) Whether the organisation or person (s) involved is/are involved in anti-state/anti-social activities and whether the persons concerned had been convicted for these or any other immoral act.

(b) Identities of the members of the executive committee of the organisation, their relationship and social status.

(c) Previous experience of the organisation in social welfare activities.

(d) Whether the organisation has its own office (Circular: Section 6.1 (d) : 1993).

If the NAB does not receive the Home Ministry's decision within the specified time, the NAB is required to send a written reminder to the Home Ministry after 30 (thirty) days (Circular: Section 6.1(d): 1993). It will then be presumed that the Ministry does not have any objection to the application for registration of the NGO concerned. The NAB is required by law to issue the letter of registration 90 days of receipt of the application. The registration remains valid for 5 years unless canceled by the state (Circular: Section 6.1(d): 1993). State retains the right to cancel the registration of an NGO. Registration can be renewed for 5 years provided NAB is satisfied with the performance of the NGO. Renewal applications should be accompanied by the constitution of the NGO, names and addresses of the members of the executive committee and minutes of the annual general meetings of the NGO and the fee for renewal or registration.

While scrutinising, the NAB has to consider whether the project contributes to socio-economic development, without duplicating existing state and non-government programmes (Circular: Section 7(1): 1993). After scrutiny, the NAB forwards the proposal to the relevant Ministry, which has to reply within 21 days. If does not, the NAB can assume that the Ministry has no objection to the project (Circular: Section 7(d) : 1993). However, if the Ministry has an objection to the project or recommends modification of the project, the arguments will have to be communicated to the NAB in detail. If it finds the objection/modification unacceptable, the NAB may approve the project after obtaining clearance from the Prime Minister's Office (Circular: Section 7(e):1993). The NAB, if necessary, can approve the project proposal after making changes and modifications. But in such a case the opinions and limitations of donor agency / agencies and relevant NGOs should be considered (Circular: Section 7(f): 1993). The NAB is required to communicate its decision within 45 days of receiving the project proposal with the requisite details (circular: Section 7(g): 1993).

[6] Any person or organisation registered as an NGO may receive or operate any foreign donation only with prior approval or permission of the state (Regulation Rules: Section 4(1): 1978). To receive / utilize foreign donations for approved projects NGOs must submit the application (through FD-2 form in triplicate) to the Director General of the NAB. The NAB issues the order to release foreign funds after consideration of the activities and budget of the NGOs approved projects, the progress and implementation of on-going projects and documents relating to receipt of foreign funds. The NAB sends copies of the order to the ERD, Bangladesh Bank (the central bank), relevant Ministries, Divisional Commissioner(s) and donor agencies for information and necessary action. In case of an approved project, to receive further installment of a foreign donation the NGO has to submit an application using form FD-2 in triplicate. Subsequently, statements of foreign donations received and spent in the previous year must be submitted on form FD-3 in triplicate. The bureau communicates its decision within 14 days of receipt of the application, after examining the annual progress report on the project.

Applications to appoint / extend the tenure of expatriates in approved projects have to be submitted by the relevant NGO to the NAB for approval or form FD-9. The NAB will ask the Home Ministry to comment within 25 days. Each proposal for appointment of expatriate personnel must be within the person-months approved by the NAB. Statements of their emoluments (even if received from outside Bangladesh) must be submitted to the NAB every year.

[7] To facilitate easy accounting, all persons or organisations registered as NGOs must receive all funds in foreign exchange through a single specified account opened in any scheduled Bank of Bangladesh which must submit statements of such funds to the central bank, i.e., The Bangladesh Bank (Regulation Rules: Section 4(4): 1978). The scheduled banks maintaining such accounts (in both foreign currency and Bangladeshi Taka) are now required to submit a statement on foreign funds to the Bangladesh Bank and the Director General of NAB every six months (Circular: Section 5(h): 1993). At present the Bangladesh Bank is supposed in its turn to

submit statements to the ERD as well as to the Director General of NAB. All NGO payments exceeding Taka 10,000 have to be made by cheque and all salaries and allowances must be paid through bank accounts (Circular: Section 5(I): 1993).

[8] The Foreign Donation (Voluntary Activities) Regulation Ordinance 1978 Section 3(1) and Section 3(3) and the Foreign Contribution (Regulation) Ordinance 1982, Section, 4(1).

[9] The Foreign Donation Regulation Act of 1978.

[10] The Exchange Control Regulation Act, 1947.

[11] The 1860 Societies Registration Act.

[12] The Government's Audit Report, 1992.

[13] Some sections of the Ordinance of 1961 may be incorporated in the Ordinance of 1978.

[14] The Bengali version of circular 1993, 'Paripatra' Section 6(KA).

[15] According to the English version of the 'Paripatra' (Section 7.1-3).

15. COMBATING CHILD LABOUR GLOBALLY: ROLE OF NON-GOVERNMENTAL ORGANISATIONS IN BANGLADESH AND NEPAL

Mojibur Rahman

BACKGROUND

It is recognised that child labour is a global concern and intervention is needed urgently both in national and international level to combat it. The number of working children between the ages of 5 and 14 in developing countries is 250 million, of whom 120 million work full time. The largest number of child workers (some 130 million or 61%) is concentrated in Asia. (ILO 1997) Being the poorest region of Asia, South Asia has the largest share of child workers in the world. Economic exploitation of children is a human rights and development issue neglected frequently. Advocacy or public awareness raising by Non-Governmental Organisations (NGOs) have taken the missing issue from the very grassroots level of the developing countries to the international level. International Labour Organisation (ILO) and United Nations Children's Fund (UNICEF) are the forefront advocates of combating child labour world wide. UN Convention on the Rights of the Child (CRC) 1989 has become a universally ratified human rights treaty and a moral code for many governments, civil society organisations and international community. New level of global concern about child labour has led governments to pass legislation against it. In South Asia, countries like Bangladesh and Nepal have signed the CRC and passed national laws against child labour. In weak states (Migdal 1988, 229) instead of multiple centres of power, land-based elite are overwhelmingly controlling state and local institutions and thwarting pro-poor development initiative because of the fear of losing status-quo. In developing countries, state actions are ordered by something other than rules e.g. the whims of the ruler, friendship or family relations, esteem, political connections or money (bribes) which characterises the "soft state" or "particularistic state". (Bolmkvist, Hans 1992, 117-150) States have policy response to protect children from economic exploitation but the operational capacity of the state institutions is very limited. In the multiplication of marginalisation and increasing vulnerability of the children in the background of state and market failure has made the NGO action inevitable. NGOs are well accepted as agent of development because of their familiarity with local people, local situation, flexible internal decision-making process and structural and operational efficiency. It is also argued that NGOs generally have a good understanding of local institutions and environment and many of them have gained confidence of the target population by reason of their familiarity with and presence at the local level. (World Bank 1983, 98)

However NGOs can not be alternative to the state rather it can be partner of the state and can play a supplementary role in development and help to break the monopoly of state and bring about institutional pluralism. NGO programmes are innovative and small-scale and termed as "small is beautiful". This has made NGOs unique in practical problem-solving, local solution of local problems which state institutions are not capable of. This paper will address the role of NGOs in South Asian states of Bangladesh and Nepal in combating child labour. International development co-operation in combating child labour will be discussed with special focus on Nordic development co-operation.

NATURE OF CHILD LABOUR IN SOUTH ASIA

Poverty along with cultural practices is often accused for child labour in developing countries. Children of lower classes and lower castes are laboured in absence of social security and safety nets of poor families in South Asia. Low growth, lack of education, poverty reproduction syndrome and marginalisation of poor are South Asian regional characteristics. In South Asia, patriarchy is the system legitimised in family, law, religion and political systems. Most of the child workers are found in farms, households and informal workshops where they are generally beyond the reach of the protective legislation and inspection. A considerable number are found in domestic services and on the streets as self-employed traders. They are in great risk of serious abuses. Child workers in dangerous occupations in South Asia ranges from the age of 5 to 14 years. Half of the South Asia's children are malnourished which is a prime cause of diseases and child mortality. (UNICEF 1998, 10) In South Asia, about 125 million children of school age are not in primary or secondary school. (Wignaraja et al 1998, 16)

In Bangladesh, situation of children is alarming where 67% children are malnourished, children out of school 18% and child labour rate under 16 is 30%. (Haq, M. 1997, 18) Cultural and religious practices against girl children in South Asia like Jari, Badeni, Dewaki and Kumari are victimising girls. A sample survey conducted by Child Workers in Nepal (CWIN) in 1990 revealed that the total workforce involved in the carpet industry within

Kathmandu district, 19% are below the age of 14 year. Children between the age of 14 to 16 years constituted 33.11% of the total workforce in the industry. (CWIN 1990) Here are some patterns of child labour in South Asia:

Urban Street Children: It is a problem in South Asia that thousands of street children live without any family and shelter in the urban streets and work near the streets or in different informal sectors in hazardous working conditions. But the problem of street children does not come from urban area itself. It comes via social exclusion and rural-urban migration.

Domestic Service: Underprivileged children work as domestic servants in rich families mainly in the urban areas out of their family environment. Girls are mainly working in domestic services in South Asia. They work as maids or cooks. There is no defined role in their work and employers do not give them free time for study or play. In many cases, employers and their family members abuse them sexually and physically. Deaths of many domestic children are unpunished. A study (1989) conducted by Save the Children-Norway (Redd Barna) shows that children are most likely to become prostitutes are housemaids, street children and children of women in prostitution. The study also claims that there are about one million sexually exploited children in Asia and working number of child prostitutes is 15,000-20,000.

Slavery: Many children in South Asia even now work in slavery or near slavery. In Nepal, bonded labour is found in some parts of the country. (INSEC 1992, 1) Despite legislation and attempts to ban the practice, selling children or giving them away in debt bondage is all too common in South Asian countries.

Sexual Exploitation: The commercial sexual exploitation of children is in the rise in global level. Sometimes poor girls are sold in prostitution and forced to work as prostitutes in many parts of South Asia. It is also a financial lure for the street girls to go to the dangerous occupation like prostitution. Trafficking of girls for sexual slavery is an acute problem there. Human rights activists estimate that up to 400 girls per month are trafficked from Bangladesh to India and Pakistan (UNICEF 1994). Nepal also has a serious problem with trafficking of girl children to work in sex trade as prostitutes in India. An estimates 4,000-5,000 Nepali girls, average age of 10-14, are annually trafficked to India. (Forum for Legal Research and Development 1994 as quoted in S. Crawford 1994, 4) Girls also work as prostitutes within Bangladesh and urban areas in Nepal. According to Human Rights Watch-Asia (1995) report 20% of Bombay's Nepali brothel population of 100,000 consists of girls under 18 years and half of them are infected with HIV.

Hazardous Occupation: In South Asia generally, children can still be found working in urban areas in hazardous industries and occupations and are exposed to chemical and biological hazards. Children work in brass-wares, glass factories, slate making, carpet weaving, and many other hazardous work. An ILO (1997) study in Bangladesh found that more than 40 types of economic activities conducted by children were hazardous. In a whole, child labour in South Asia is found to be intolerable by international standards:

- child work similar to slavery
- forced and bonded labour of children
- commercial sexual exploitation
- work exposing children to health and safety hazards

It is estimated that children employed in export industries in the world represent only a small fraction of the total problem of child labour in the world -- estimated less than 5% (ILO & UNICEF 1997); the vast majority of children are engaged in production for domestic consumption, rather than in export sector. In this situation, the call for trade barrier on countries have child labour products by some developed countries is similar to call for take away the comparative advantage enjoyed by developing countries in international trade. Rather the issue should be dealt as a human rights and development issue with human solidarity.

CHILD LABOUR A GLOBAL CHALLENGE

A vigorous campaign by NGOs and the United Nations system has taken the issue in the global agenda. CRC of 1989 is the moral charter of rights of the children recognised by international community. The convention has been ratified by 187 countries, covering 97 per cent of the worlds children. (Fallon & Tzannatos 1998, 6) The creation of International Programme for Elimination of Child Labour (IPEC) of ILO in 1992 was one of the biggest step in international response to the problem. World Congress against Commercial Sexual Exploitation of Children held in Stockholm in 1996 is another hope for exploited and potentially exploited children. IPEC is working to eliminate child labour world wide by strengthening capability of individual countries to deal with the problem. The number of IPEC donors have increased to 14[1]. It has programmes in 27 countries including Bangladesh and Nepal. It has close link with local and international NGOs.

---

[1]IPEC donors- Australia, Belgium, Canada, Denmark, European Commission, France, Germany, Italy, Luxembourg, the Netherlands, Spain, Switzerland, United Kingdom and the United States.

The World Summit on Social Development-WSSD held in 1995 is one of the cornerstone of the rights of the children. The summit called for a 20/20 initiative in social development. In Copenhagen approximately 2800 separate organisations came together in an NGO Forum 95. Many NGO representatives were also allowed to attend the government summit. Later, Amsterdam and Oslo conference on child labour and the Global March Against Child Labour by civil society organisations has made the issue explicit to the people of the world. The UN Convention on the Rights of the Child affirms the rights of the children:

> ...to education, self-expression, and freedom from exploitative work, children are not adults, their fundamental right is to childhood itself. (Fyfe, A. 1993, 5)

In Finnish development co-operation, children's rights are indivisible and state supports development efforts of underprivileged children in developing countries. The government states that children's rights are universal and violation of these rights cannot be justified by appealing to cultural differences, national characteristics or tradition in the four corners of the globe. (Ministry of Foreign Affairs of Finland 1998)

Inter-Parliamentary Union (IPU) Final Declaration on Democracy highlighted on the combating of child labour. It called on states to (1997) *... reduce child labour through compulsory primary education for boys and girls, including substantial investment in education involving civil society and local government.*

Recognising children's perspective in development co-operation is an urgent need as economic exploitation of children is a global human rights and development issue. The idea of policy dialogue and capacity building with strengthening the NGO capacities and networks of international and local human rights organisations are fundamental to new human rights strategy of OECD countries. (DAC 1996) Donors are suggesting the World Bank's (1990) three-pronged approach to poverty reduction strategy for developing countries which include broad-based growth, investing in people and safety nets. Logically, working children should get priority in their right to development through local, national and international initiative. For many years, NGOs have argued that donors should make clear how much of their ODA to education and health goes to primary education and health care. (ICVA, Eurostep, ActionAid 1995, 16)

Deacon (1997, 200) has shown the model of global social policy where welfare failure and social neglect by regimes put the mass in insecurity and NGOs play a vital role amidst state and market failure. As Southern people's movements are directed towards a sustainable development and NGOs are playing a catalyst role in development,

Northern NGOs have a very important role to play by supporting Southern NGOs vis-a-vis Southern peoples movement. Malena, C. (1995, 11) suggests that ...the role of Northern NGOs, should be to assist Southern NGOs in building their organisational capacity, thus promoting the establishment and development of viable indigenous institutions and structures which will sustain the development process on a long term basis.

NORDIC DEVELOPMENT CO-OPERATION, NGOS AND CHILDREN'S PERSPECTIVE

In the wake of globalisation, Structural Adjustment Programme (SAP) came in force and some vulnerable groups like children are the worst effected group in this global tendency. In 1980s, UNICEF criticised the World Bank's SAP for worsening living conditions of the poorest groups, a judgement which was supported by Nordic countries and the Netherlands and Canada. It is a positive approach which giving social tools to protect human rights of children as human rights include not only political and civil rights but also economic, social and cultural rights and right to development. Northern NGOs have co-operation with Southern NGOs through consulting, lobbying, networking, overseas activities, publishing and research activities in the concerned field. In 1987, UNICEF used terms like "adjustment with a Human Face" -- putting importance on children's demand for education and development. There is a global network of stakeholders in combating child labour. There are local and Nordic NGOs and NGOs from other OECD countries working in Bangladesh and Nepal for example. Bilateral co-operation, co-operation through multilateral agencies like UNICEF, ILO, UNESCO, UNDP, WHO and co-operation with NGOs through the development co-operation are some forms of development assistance. Nordic input into multilateral agencies like UNICEF and UNDP constitutes nearly 30 per cent. (The Nordic Way 1995, 37) The role of NGOs has been emphasised by all Nordic countries in the protection of human rights. For example, roughly a quarter of Sweden's total development assistance is allocated through NGOs (The Nordic Way 1995, 23) Denmark supports human rights packages involving Danish NGOs and supporting local human rights organisations in recipient countries. (DANIDA 1991, 85) With the exception of Finland after recession, the Nordic countries are the top of the DAC countries in providing aid above the UN target of 0.7% of their GDP. Finland made rapid progress during the 1980s and in reaching 0.8% in 1991, then fell to 0.3% by 1994. Yet, the Nordic countries, as a whole, gave 0.8% in 1994 while the average for DAC countries was only 0.3%. (UM 1995, 8)

Basic education both formal and non-formal are important for human capacity development which should be given priority in development aid. Aid in other social sectors like health care, water and sanitation, family planning and nutrition can be supportive to basic education to combat vulnerability of the children. Like-minded Countries[2] give more human priorities in bilateral aid comparing to other OECD countries. During 1991/92-1993, a number of education donors like Finland, the Netherlands, Norway and Sweden witnessed significant decline in education support. (Buchert, L. 1995, 16-7)

NGOs are considered as effective because of their poverty focus, innovation and flexibility. Aid through NGO channel is a significant component of development co-operation in the present aid policies of Nordic countries. Over the past two decades, official donors have increased their funding of NGO development projects. (ODI 1995) In recent years 10% and 15% of aid to developing countries from OECD countries was channelled through NGOs. (ODI 1996)

In 1998, Finland was supposed to channel 20% more funds to NGOs development assistance than 1997. Most of the operations concentrate on health, education and in other social sectors. (Development Today 1998) In Finnish development co-operation policy by decision-in-principle mentioned by the cabinet in 1996, assistance channelled through NGOs will be increased 10-15 per cent of the budget for development co-operation proper and state will encourage NGOs to participate in bilateral projects and humanitarian aid. Finland has committed itself to raise it's level of aid to 0.4% of GNP by the year 2000. (Ministry of Foreign Affairs 1998, 6)

A recent opinion survey on "Finnish Attitude to Aid" prepared by Taloustutkimus Oy and Ministry of Foreign Affairs suggests that Finns prioritise aid in promoting human rights, democracy and social justice by 40% of the sample. According to the survey, respecting human rights should be the most important condition for aid. (Development Today 1998)

In the beginning of 1990s, the share of Norwegian bilateral aid to NGOs was 25% with upward trend. (Tvedt, T. 1995, i) According to the Norwegian Agency for Development Co-operation's (NORAD) Annual Report 1996, in the 1990s there has been increasing emphasis on the importance of basic education and primary health care services in development co-operation. (NORAD 1996, 14)

---

[2] Nordic countries, Canada and the Netherlands

Education is perhaps the most important investment in social development because educated people are more productive and therefore contribute more to country's growth. Poverty is the primary cause of child labour in developing countries. Children from the poorest families go to work because of poverty. A study by UNDP (1992, 23) suggests that land ownership and household income are two most important factors which determines the participation of children in school in developing countries. Social structure and institutional neglect to the poor are responsible for poverty, hunger and episodes of famine in the world. Schools represent the most important means of drawing children away from labour market.

According to ILO (1995) , the single most effective way to stem the flow of school age children into abusive forms of employment is to extend and improve schooling so that it will attract and retain them. Working children or potential working children have little or no chance to receive education because of the poverty of their families. Parents do not understand the importance of schooling for their children from their own experience. Parental education plays a large role in determining child's schooling and employment (Tienda 1979, 370-391).

From the very old times, schools were highly honoured where the children of upper classes were diligent students. The idea of school was to form harmonious personalities with balanced intellectual, aesthetic and physical development of the learners. This aristocratic conception was nurtured for centuries by imperial, royal and feudal societies. The practice structurally dedicated to cultivating a selective education and it is still remaining in certain educational systems of modern age. Developing countries have not got out of the mentality which divides the society according to class. This selective educational system does not recognise the rights of the underprivileged children in education and make democracy and social justice difficult. Traditional schools in developing countries create some memorising students to be the civil servants and professionals related to money and power (Rahman, Mojibur 1998).

Children from well off families enjoy the right to education which furthers social inequality. State supported educational system does not care for the underprivileged children and thwarts their endeavour to participate in schools. For certain groups, exclusion from the educational system is often a form of political oppression, and if they gain access, educational programmes often ignore their needs (Boonpala, Bose & Haspels 1997).

To practice democracy in the state level requires the democratisation of the educational system with adoption and implementation of the

Universal Primary Education (UPE). All children must be guaranteed the practical possibility of receiving basic education, full time if possible, in other forms if necessary. Bangladesh and Nepal have signed the World Declaration on Education for All. Both governments have created a National Plan of Action and set ambitious targets for primary education. With international co-operation, in 1993, Bangladesh introduced compulsory primary education for children of relevant age group. In the government schools, there is no tuition fees, text books along with the required stationary articles are provided to the students free of cost. (Planning Commission of Bangladesh 1990-95)

But all these incentives could not ensure full educational participation by the entire primary age group population. Non-enrolment and drop-out rate of children in school is still high. In Nepal, the net enrolment for boys and girls in the elementary school is 64% and 31%. (National Planning Commission of Nepal 1992) Those non-starters and drop-outs are the potential illiterate adults and run risk of vulnerability if there is no alternative or supplementary education.

The education children get from school is alien to them who find it no solution to the problems of the environment in which they must transform to achieve their development. The problem of educational system in developing countries are:

- bureaucratisation and centralisation
- lack of relevance in working life
- lack of pluralism in educational provision
- lack of social mobilisation and community participation
- lowest enrolment of girls in school system
- ignore the special needs of working children and disabled.

The challenge of education to developing countries is to shun the spirit of bygone days and revive their commitment to learning. SAARC countries have made joint strategy for pro-poor planning where priorities include:

- food security
- literacy and primary education
- primary health care
- protection of children. (Wignaraja et al 1998, 289)

NGOs IN NON-FORMAL EDUCATION IN BANGLADESH AND NEPAL

The social movements in developing countries have attracted growing interest of development thinkers. International conventions on human rights of children can not ensure the rights of the child without institutional programming with flexibility and innovation in the operational level. There is a need for transformation of cultural, social, economic and political structures in developing countries concerning children. A study conducted in 1978 by INNOTECH (UNESCO-UNICEF) concluded that life skills are valuable for all children to learn whether or not they have left school at an early age. (Baine 1988, 19) In the experience of the'grassroots based women NGO 'Saptagram' in Bangladesh, the women of adult literacy programme asked the movement to provide education for their children. (Guttman, C. 1994, 14) In formal schools, there is a traditional divorce between formal and vocational education which impoverishes the underprivileged children. Mismatches between education and occupation and widening gap between the formal schooling and it's accomplishment has created educational democracy difficult. This mismatching between school and society reminds the need for alternative or complementary education. The "diploma disease" (Dore 1976) or "credentialism" (Berg 1971) is a reflection of a manipulation of the educational system by market forces. Instead of being an equaliser, the school creates class differences and polarises society. To avoid this polarisation, some critic like Ivan Illich called for "deschooling of society". In their action, some NGOs have focused on non-formal basic education in a reasonable cost with maintaining relevance, equity and efficiency. Non-Formal Education (NFE) is organised by NGOs for out-of-school and drop-out children where formal education have failed to address their problem because of their timing, hierarchy. In developing countries, NFE is a neglected form of education but in some developed countries it is flourishing and playing a wide variety of roles i.e. fulfilling peoples need. (Carron & Carr-Hill 1991, 11-2) Realising the importance of NGOs as partners of development, World Bank's South Asia region has formal and informal consultative group with a number of concerned NGOs. (Fallon & Tzannatos 1998, viii) Governments of Bangladesh and Nepal recognise the role of non-formal education initiated by NGOs as complementary to the goal of UPE. NGOs put special emphasis on girls education which is a key component of protecting them from violence and help to build a sustainable future for them. NGOs are combining education and training for children from literacy and health education. NGOs in Bangladesh like Bangladesh Rural Advancement Committee (BRAC), Underprivileged Children's Education Programme (UCEP), Rädda Barnen (Save the Children-Sweden), Red Barnet (Save the Children -Denmark), Suomen Vapaa Ulkolähetys (Finnish Free Foreign Mission), Terre Des Hommes (Netherlands), Norwegian Association of the Blind, Save the Children Fund- Australia are working to protect children's right. In Nepal, Child

Workers in Nepal Concerned Center- CWIN, Underprivileged Children's Education Programme (UCEP), Finnish NGO in Development Co-operation 'Taksvärkki', Norwegian Association of the Blind, Nepal Children's Organisation-NCO, Redd Barna (Save the Children-Norway), USC Nepal (Canada), Save the Children-USA are working to protect children's rights.

After the ban on child labour in garment industries in Bangladesh by US Harkins Bill, the affected children were provided NFE initiated under the agreement among UNICEF, ILO and Bangladesh Garments Manufacturers and Exporting Association (BGMEA) and under the agreement, BRAC and Gono Sahajjo Sangstha (GSS), two prominent Bangladeshi NGOs are engaged in educating children under the project. BRAC is operating some 256 schools for child workers in some areas like Dhaka, Narayanganj, Chittagong and Gazipur.[3] UCEP is having programmes in Bangladesh and Nepal. It is working with national and international partners in protecting working children. It has general literacy as well as technical and vocational training in the field of general mechanical, auto mechanical, drafting and printing press, tailoring and electrical training. The NGO works mainly with the working children aged from 12 to 18 years and UCEP- Nepal has special focus on children from remote region, ethnic minority and weaker sex. In Bangladesh, Rädda Barnen is providing courses for training of staffs of the International Save the Children Alliance, police officers, trainers of police academy and refreshers course for training for trainers about the rights of children. (Rädda Barnen 1996, 3) The NGO is supporting local NGOs such as Bangladesh Shishu Adhikar Forum (BSAF) and National Forum of Organizations Working with the Disabled (NFOWD).

BRAC's NFPE which was created in 1985 has attracted donor attention and co-operation. It is working with NFE for children of the age group for 8-10 and 11-16. It has mobilised children from poor families in education and 70% of the attendants are girls, participating in three-year primary education programme. Over 8000 single teacher schools were projected to be increased to 50,000 by 1995. The drop-out rate students over the three year cycle is less than 2% compared to over 60% in public sector schools. (Wignaraja et al 1998, 54-5) After completion of the BRAC schooling, children can successfully attend in the public schools in upper grade. The system is introduced for three-year education because, in that

---

[3]Information sent from BRAC's Non-Formal Primary Education (NFPE) Programme, Dhaka, Bangladesh on 29.03.1998.

level of education, most of the children drop-out of the school. The success of BRAC schooling are:

- less than 5% drop-out
- 90% graduating from NFPE gain admittance to grade IV in formal schools
- 75% girl enrolment

The success of BRAC's NFE programme puts pressure on the public schools for more efficiency. Characteristics of BRAC programme are:

- three year curricula
- 8-10 and 11-16 year age group
- complementary dealing with drop-outs and non-starters
- school timing suitable for children's needs
- need-based curricula
- parents in school management

Prevention of child exploitation project in Nepal is running by both local and international NGOs. Local NGOs like CWIN and NCO are in the forefront in this action. The project is supported by Redd Barna, Australian Agency for International Development, Save the children Fund-UK and the UNICEF national committees of Finland, Germany and the Netherlands. Advocacy for the children's rights by NGOs in Nepal is a success. A 150-member NGO children's rights advocacy network were established. (UNICEF 1996) A number of NGOs are working with child prostitutes, street children and children in prison. IPEC programme in Nepal has partnership for implementing projects with local NGOs. NGO initiated programmes mobilise local people against exploitation of children. In the case of child trafficking, they have initiated mobilising local police, teachers, youth and community leaders to play an active role in monitoring trafficking movements in Nepal. NGO activities include various types of alternatives for children including prevention, NFE, skill training, personal development, family income generation, participation, awareness raising and community strengthening programmes. Taksvärkki is carrying out a project in Nepal in co-operation with CWIN to improve the possibilities of street children and child workers of Kathmandu for education. The project include skill development for underprivileged girl children, socialisation for street children and shelter for children at risk.

CONCLUSION

NGOs run their projects or programmes in micro level and some of the South Asian NGOs have yielded good impact on the life of working children by providing need based education. Successful NGO models tell the world that it is possible to provide education for working children effectively to fight economic exploitation. The potential of NGOs should be used by co-ordination among NGOs who are working in the same field with more international co-operation. Successful NGO experience can be used in national level programme concerning working children. Local and international co-operation is necessary to use NGO expertise in protecting underprivileged childhood from economic exploitation.

REFERENCES

Baine, David (1988): *Handicapped Children in Developing Countries: Assessment, Curriculum and Instruction.* Edmonton: University of Alberta Press.

Berg, Ivar (1971): *Education and Jobs: The Great Training Robbery.* Boston: Beacon Press.

Bolmkvist, Hans (1992): The Soft State: Making Policy in Different Context. In Doglas Ashford (ed) *history and Context in Comparative Public Policy.* Pittsburgh: University of Pittsburgh Press.

Boonpala, P. & Bose, C. & Haspel, N. (1997): *Educational Strategies for the Prevention and Elimination of Child Labour: Synthesis report of 13 Country Studies on the Mobilization of Teachers, Educators and Their Organizations in Combating Child Labour.* Unpublished Manuscript. Geneva: IPEC & ILO.

Buchert, Lene (1995): *Recent Trends in Education Aid: Towards a Classification of Policies.* Paris: UNESCO-International Institute of educational Planning.

Carron, Gabriel & Carr-Hill, R. A. (1991): *Non-Formal Education: Information and Planning Issues.* IIEP Research Report No. 90. Paris: International Institute of Educational Planning.

Crawford, Susan (1994): *Child Labour in Asia: A Review of the Literature.* Princeton: UNICEF Regional Office for South Asia.

CWIN (1990): *Lost Childhood: Survey Research on Street Children of Kathmandu.* Kathmandu: Child Labour in Nepal (CWIN) Concerned Centre.

DAC (1996): DAC strategic document on *"Shaping the 21st Century: The Contribution of Development Cooperation"* adopted in the 34th high level meeting of DAC, held on 6-7 May, 1996.

DANIDA (1991): Human Rights and Democracy in Danish Development Cooperation. In Krause & Rosas (eds) *Development Cooperation and Process Towards Democracy.* Helsinki: FINNIDA.

Deacon, Bob et al (1997): *Global Social Policy- International Organizations and the Future of Welfare.* London: Sage Publications.

Development Today (1998): *Development Today,* Vol. Viii, No. 5-6, April 21, 1998

Development Today (1998): Vol. Viii, No. 2, February 1998, "Development Survey: Finnish Attitude to Aid on the Upswing"

Dore, Ronald (1976): The Diploma Disease: Education, Qualification and Development. London: Allen & Unwin.

Fallon, P. & Tzannatos, Z. (1998): *Child Labour: Issues and Direction for the World Bank.* Washington, D.C. : The World Bank.

Fyfe, Alec (1993): *Child Labour: A Guide to Project Design.* Geneva: ILO.

Guttman, Cynthia (1994): *In Our Own Hands: The Story of Saptagram: A Women's Self-Reliance and Education Movement in Bangladesh.* Paris: UNESCO.

Haq, Mahbub Ul (1997): *Human Development in South Asia 1997.* New York: Oxford University Press.

Human Rights Watch-Asia (1995): *Rape for Profit: Trafficking of Nepali Girls and Women to India's Brothels.* Human Rights Watch-Asia

ICVA, Eurostep/ActionAid (1995): *The Reality of Aid: An Independent Review of International Aid.* London: ActionAid.

ILO & UNICEF (1997): *Document presented by ILO and UNICEF in International Conference on Child Labour in Oslo,* 27-30 October, 1997

ILO (1996): *Child Labour: What is to be Done?* ILO

ILO (1997): *Child Labour in Asia.* ILO

ILO (1997): *World of Work,* No. 19, March 1997, 'New Weapons Against Child Trafficking in Asia'. ILO

INSEC (1992): *Bonded Labour in Nepal Under Kamaiya System.* Kathmandu: Informal Sector Service Centre.

Inter-Parliamentary Union (1997): Bulletin 2/97, July-December 1997. *Inter-Parliamentary Union*

Malena, C. (1995): Relations Between Northern and Southern Non-Governmental Development Organizations. In: *Canadian Journal of Development Studies.* Vol.xvi, No. 1, 1995. Ottawa: Canadian Association for the Study of International Development.

Migdal, Joel S. (1988): *Strong Societies and Weak States: State-Society Relations and State Capacities in the Third world.* Princeton: Princeton University Press.

Ministry of Foreign Affairs (1996): *Decision-in-Principle on Finland's Development Co-operation.* The Cabinet 12.9.1996. Helsinki: Department of international Development Co-operation.

Ministry for Foreign Affairs of Finland (1998): *Finland Takes Children's Side.* Helsinki: Ministry for Foreign Affairs of Finland

National Planning Commission of Nepal (1992): *National Planning*

Commission of Nepal, 1992. Kathmandu: National Planning Commission of Nepal

NORAD (1996): *Annual Report 1996.* Oslo: Royal Ministry of Foreign Affairs.

ODI (1995): *ODI Briefing Paper 1995(4)*, NGOs and Official Donors.

ODI (1996): *ODI Briefing Paper 1996(2)*, The Impact of NGO Development Projects

Planning Commission of Bangladesh (1990-95): *The Fourth Five Year Plan (1990-95).* Dhaka: Planning Commission of Bangladesh

Rahman, Mojibur (1998): *Globalization, Development Cooperation and Human Rights of Children in Least Developed Countries: South Asia in Context.* Paper Presented in the Annual Conference of Norwegian Association for Development research-NFU on "Development Ethics". Oslo, 5-6 June, 1998.

Rädda Barnen (1996): *Annual Report 1996.* Dhaka: Swedish Save the Children Bangladesh.

The Nordic Way (1995): *Social Summit Special.* Copenhagen: DANIDA.

Tienda, M. (1979): Economic Activity of Children in Peru: Labor Force Behavior in Rural and Urban Contexts. In *Rural Sociology.*

Tvedt, Terje (1995): *NGOs as a Channel in Development Aid: The Norwegian System.* Oslo: Royal Ministry of Foreign Affairs.

UM (1995): *Suomen Kehitysyhteistyön Perustilastot.* Helsinki: Ulkoasiainministeriö, Kehitysyhteistyöosasto, Painatuskeskus Oy.

UNDP (1992): *Human Development in Bangladesh: Local Action Under National Constraints.* Dhaka: UNDP Human Development Institute.

UNICEF (1996): *Country Programme Recommendation on Nepal.* UNICEF

UNICEF (1998): *The State of World's Children 1998.* New York: Oxford University Press.

UNICEF/Rosa (1994): *Report on South Asian Girl Child in Especially Difficult Circumstances.* UNICEF

Wignaraja, P. & Sirivardana, Susil (1998): *Readings on Pro-Poor Planning through Social Mobilization in South Asia. Vol. 1.* The Strategic Option for Poverty Alleviation. New Delhi: Vikas Publishing House (Pvt) Ltd.

World Bank (1983): *Bangladesh: Selected Issues in Rural Employment.* Washington, D.C.: World Bank.

World Bank (1990): *World Development Report 1990.* Washington, D. C.: World Bank

16. GOVERNMENT-NGO COLLABORATION: A STUDY OF SELECTED HEALTH SECTOR PROJECTS IN BANGLADESH

Salahuddin Aminuzzaman, Afroza Begum & F. R. M. Mortuza Huq

INTRODUCTION

NGOs have become a focal point of attention for development thinkers and practitioners since the 1980s. There has been a significant world wide growth of NGOs, and their capacity to contribute to the development process has expanded considerably (Korten 1991). One recent trend in development management is the emergence of Government Organisations (GOs) and Non-government Organisations (NGOs) collaboration. In fact, two-fold realisation have steered the GO-NGO collaboration in developing countries. The governments are reckoning with the fact that they have to incorporate in their operational modalities the features which account largely for NGO success. On the other hand, the NGOs have increasingly recognised that they cannot operate their programmes in isolation from the extensive government delivery mechanism and institutional framework. (Bhattacharia & Ahmed 1995)

GO-NGO RELATIONSHIP: PREMISE AND RATIONALE

GO-NGO relations vary enormously from country to country and from regime to regime. In some situations, NGOs are viewed as clear opponents of the GOs and their relations are no less than hostile. In other cases, GOs and NGOs are found sharing similar goals and work closely with each other. Between the two extremes, there are governments which may tolerate the NGO sector without being particularly supportive or which might ally themselves with certain NGOs while opposing others. Given the enormous heterogeneity of the NGO sector, a government's relationship with any individual organisation depends greatly upon that organisation's specific activities, purpose, ideology, institutional or personal ties. (Maleha 1995)

There are two sets of opinions about the collaboration between GOs and NGOs (Fernandez 1987). One group holds that NGOs should not collaborate formally in programmes sponsored by GOs and therefore should not receive funds directly from GOs; to do so NGOs would lose their independence and voluntarism. The other group holds that NGOs have a role to play in GO programmes aimed at poverty alleviation, a role which is essential to the success of the programmes and which the government cannot provide. Thus, GOs should support the NGOs to enable them to fulfil their objectives.

The rationale for GO-NGO collaboration can be argued on the following grounds

Collaboration ensures poor's participation: Participation of the poor in the development process requires sensitising the poor through consciousness raising and functional education resulting in their capacity building. NGOs have proven their ability to demonstrate on how the capacity of the poor can be developed. GO-NGO collaboration also ensures the accessibility of the poor to the public services.

Collaboration creates the effective demand of the poor for public services: Many GO programmes are supply-oriented e.g. immunisation programme, credit delivery programme etc. The poor are mostly deprived of these supplies, as they fail to make effective demand as well as there exists no suitable receiving mechanism at the grass-roots level. NGOs can help the poor in this respect by organising them, by developing their awareness and by creating their income opportunities through various employment generation programmes. Thus NGOs can help the poor to make effective demand for public services. On the other hand, NGOs can also help the GOs by sharing their experience and local knowledge at the grass-root level. GO-NGO collaboration therefore would develop institutional means to provide the facilities of public services to the poor at the grass-root level.

Collaboration ensures to utilise the knowledge and ability of both the counterparts: NGOs in the developing countries have acquired rich experience and meaningful insights in programme planning and implementation, training, monitoring and evaluation of the programmes. GO-NGO collaboration creates an opportunity for GO institutions to utilise the experience of the NGOs and at the same time it also provides the scope for the NGOs to expand their programmes on large scale.

Collaboration ensures the country-wide expansion of successful programmes: Though NGOs in the developing countries have experienced with some highly successful programmes, they can hardly be able to replicate these programmes on large scale basis because of their limits of institutional and resource absorptive capacity. GO-NGO collaboration generates the GO support towards the successful programmes of the NGOs to expand, faster and widen the scope of the successful programme on nation wide basis.

Collaboration creates a new working system in the development scenario: GO-NGO collaboration may contribute towards the emergence of a system of organisations having functional specialisation which will ensure removal of overlap, foster mutual help and assistance, supplement each others' work and facilitate resolution of conflicts.

Collaboration ensures pluralism: In pursuing the goals of national development an important and essential factor is pluralism. Along with the GOs, the NGO sector is considered as an important part of a pluralistic society. GO-NGO collaboration ensures pluralism which helps to expand the growth of NGO sector to share important common goals with the GOs.

Collaboration ensures the utilisation of the potentials of all Sectors: With a view to attain national development it is very much essential to utilise the potentials and advantages of all the sectors. Though the government & GOs have the responsibility for determining the general policy directions for the national development but it is not possible for the government alone to bring about sustainable improvements in the lives of the poor. The extensive network of NGOs specially at the grass-root level can help GOs to tackle the nation's vast development needs.

Collaboration ensures cost effectiveness: The high cost effectiveness of NGO projects is often quoted as another reason for collaboration. This is certainly true in cases where NGOs have built up local structures which official agencies coming new to the field, would be obliged to create for themselves.

Both GOs and NGOs enjoy various advantages from collaboration (Ferrington & Bebbington 1993). The following table represent a general summary of the benefits that both of the counterparts enjoy from collaborative programmes.

Table 1. Advantages of Collaborative Programme

NGOs perspective	GOs perspective
1. Gaining access to research expertise and technological resources in GO.	1. Helps gaining access to the technical innovations and strategies of NGOs.
2. Helps to scale - up NGO generated innovations through the GO apparatus.	2. NGOs can help implementing public policy and monitoring and coordinating grass root activities.
3. Greater and easy access to GO agencies.	3. NGOs can train the field level GO staff to motivate and innovate participatory people oriented approach.
4. Create opportunity to advocate and motivate GO staff to be more people oriented.	4. NGOs can be used as sub-contractors of GO projectsin the remote places.
5. Provide means of exercising pressure over GO agencies, to urge them to reorient their policies.	5. GO can use NGOs to mobilize people more effectively.

However there are some practical problems in the process of GO-NGO collaboration. These problems are:

Problem of autonomy: GO-NGO collaboration in many cases challenges NGOs' functional autonomy. By engaging in co-ordinated programmes, NGOs have to surrender a certain degree of autonomy over their own actions and the external factors tend to influence their operational strategies.

Problem for diversity and mutual mistrust: There are considerable diversity among NGOs as regards to their philosophies, objectives, mode and scale of operation. GOs are similarly diverse in the development objectives they pursue. Besides GO-NGOs have very different working approaches. These diversities create numerous functional problems in the collaboration projects. In many cases both GOs and NGOs tend to mistrust each other in terms of sharing credit and outcome of the project.

Unfavourable and ambiguous policies: In most of the developing countries in spite of policy pronouncements, still there are some in built contradictions in various laws, procedural approaches in GO-NGO collaboration. GO-NGO collaboration are constrained by the fact that the respective roles and responsibilities of the collaborating bodies are not clearly spelled out in the agreements of collaboration which leads to serious problem at the implementation stage.

Bureaucratic populism: The more obvious obstacles steam from bureaucratic populism as GOs tend to perceive NGOs as a threat or competitor (Ferrington & Bebbington 1993).

Preconditions for Successful Collaboration:

GO-NGO collaboration is a felt need of the present time. For successful collaboration, there are some preconditions (Paul, S 1991). They are: **a.** Openness and willingness for collaboration from both sides; **b.** mutual trust and respect; **c.** Favourable GO policy; **d.** Favourable socio-economic and political environments; **e.** Acceptance of autonomy and independence; **f.** Pluralism of NGO opinion and positions; **g.** Adequate channels of institutional communication; **h.** Mutual learning process, training and support; **i.** Transparency of activities, and Accountability of concerned GO and NGO staff.

NGOs IN BANGLADESH

Inhuman sufferings of people and a massive destruction of the physical infra-structure and the economy brought by the War of Liberation in early 1970s called for immediate relief and rehabilitation interventions. Government of Bangladesh (GOB) had to face a Herculean tasks of renewal and reconstruction of the war torn economy. But the GOB neither had the capacity nor had the appropriate institutional mechanism to address to the volume and diversity of such enormous problems single handed. At that point of time a large number of international NGOs and voluntary organisations extended their helping hands to assist Bangladesh (Aminuzzaman 1993). Besides a few national organisations were established during that period as a spontaneous responses from a number of committed people, which are at present well-known leading NGOs in Bangladesh such as BRAC, *Gonoshasthaya Kendra, Proshika, Nijera Kori,* etc.

Certain objective conditions has fostered the emergence and growth of NGOs in Bangladesh. Following section makes an overview of the endogenous and exogenous conditions / factors.

a. Tradition of Voluntary Activities: Voluntary undertakings by individuals or groups intending to serve and benefit the people have been in vogue for centuries in this country. With the changing social structures and consequent changes in beliefs, practices and social relations, the concept of voluntarism has marked a radical swing along a direction that involves professionalism, invites specialisation and invokes formal management structures, which can be seen in contemporary NGOs operation in Bangladesh. In other words, volunteering is a part of the culture and religion of the people of Bangladesh ((Huda 1987).

b. Dissatisfaction of Donor Agencies: One of the main reasons for the rapid growth of NGOs in Bangladesh is a growing dissatisfaction of donor agencies with public organisations which are considered to be slow, rigid, hierarchic and inefficient in delivering public services (Aminuzzaman 1993). On the other hand, support from bilateral and multilateral agencies for NGOs in Bangladesh has steadily increased as a reflection of the perceived capacity and effectiveness of the NGOs in working with the poor (ADB 1992).

c. Unsuccessful Governmental Efforts: Many of the macro-policy-reforms, made by GOB with a view to benefiting the poor, have failed to achieve desired successes from time to time, due to the non-existence of appropriate institutions to execute such reforms at the grass-root level . The success of NGOs lies with their capacity to deal creatively with situations because of their small size and their concentration on a limited number of activities. Thus where GOB fail to achieve the desired success, NGOs can play there an important role in complementing the governmental efforts (Huda 1987). The emergence of NGOs in Bangladesh is directly related to the failure of the government to meet the hopes and aspirations of the people.

d. An Increase in Foreign Aid: The mushrooming growth of NGOs in Bangladesh is also due to the increase in foreign aid and humanitarian help to cope with many natural disasters that Bangladesh often experience. Foreign funding is considered as a lucrative opportunity to resources for the NGOs.

f. Successful in Sectoral Development: NGO activities have virtually grown into a movement in Bangladesh. NGOs play a very significant role in the nation's development process. They have assumed a vital role in sectors such as poverty alleviation, family planning, gender issue of women in development, health education / awareness, rural development, improvement of infrastructure and in environment protection. In public sector these areas of activities though incorporated in national plans and programmes have received scanty attention and resource allocation at the implementation level (Shelly 1992).

NUMBER OF NGOS IN BANGLADESH

The world of NGOs in Bangladesh is inadequately documented (Shelly 1992). As the existing literature on NGOs is scatter and incomplete, there are various estimates as to the total number of NGOs in Bangladesh. There are still no official statistics of the number of NGOs in Bangladesh. As a matter of fact, different agencies of the government like the

Department of Social Service; Joint Stock Company, Department of Women Affairs, Department of Youth Development ; Department of Family Planning, Department of Non- Formal Education give registration to the NGOs separately. These departments have independent authority to give registration to the NGOs. According to the recent statement made to the National Parliament by the Minister of Commerce and Industries the number of non-government organisations (NGOs) registered with different government departments is about 20000. The Minister further informed the house that there are 1237 NGOs which are involved in implementing foreign aided projects (Daily Star, Friday 13, March). Though the members of NGOs are quite big, but a survey undertaken by the ADB reports up to November 1988 about two-thirds of the total were found to be inactive (ADB 1989). One estimate claims that NGOs operate in more than 78 percent of the total villages of the country involving over 3.5 million families as beneficiaries of their work (ADAB 1994).

HEALTH SECTOR NGOS IN BANGLADESH

Though there are about 20000 NGOs in Bangladesh, only a selected few are directly involved in health related projects or programmes. According to the data published by Voluntary Health Services Society (VHSS)[1] there are 198 NGOs both international and local that are involved in health projects.

It is to be noted here that though there are about 198 registered NGOs in health sector, but not all of these are specialised health care NGO. Most of these NGOs have regular development projects catering the need of the so-called disadvantaged groups and the poor. In addition to their regular programmes, these NGOs have some health education and health related community mobilisation programmes. In most cases the NGO programmes include awareness regarding immunisation, family planning practices, campaign for safe drinking water, and basic health education. With exception of a few, most of these NGOs do not have direct health care facilities and or programme interventions for their respective clientele groups.

---

[1] The VHSS is the national coalition of the health sector NGOs in Bangladesh. It is a coordinating and support service agency for the NGOs actively involved in health throughout Bangladesh. VHSS has come a long way since its beginning in 1978 when total number of members was only 28, which stands to 198 as of date. VHSS maintains links with government, donor and the NGOs.

Table 2. Growth of Health Project NGOs in Bangladesh

Year of Establishment	Number of NGOs	Percentage	Cum %
Before 1971*	14	7.33%	7.33%
1971 - 1975	23	12.04%	19.37%
1976 - 1980	32	16.75%	36.13%
1981 - 1985	60	31.41%	67.54%
1986 - 1990	38	19.90%	87.43%
1991 - 1995	22	11.52%	98.95%
1996 - to Date	2	1.05%	100.00%
Total	192	100%	100.00%

Data for 8 NGOs were not available

Table 1. presents an overall picture of the growth of health care NGOs in Bangladesh. It clearly reveals that these NGOs emerged significantly after 1980s - more than half i.e., 51.3 percent of these NGOs came into operation during the period of 1981 - 1990. During the next five to six years yet another 12.5 percent of these NGOs initiated their operations.

This growth pattern shows the increasing concern of the international donor community regarding the health sector and their emphasis for integrating the NGO sector in health management and delivery system in Bangladesh. About 42 percent of the Health Sector NGOs are based in the capital city and other major metropolis. Rest 51 percent of these NGOs are either based in district towns (29.75%) and in small Thana Towns (23.56%).

Table 2. and 3. give an overview of the coverage of programme areas and the beneficiaries of the programmes run by the NGOs. 71.6 percent of these NGOs cover up to 10 Thana[2] by their respective projects. An in-depth look into the table further reveals that programme intervention of 93 percent of these NGOs are confined to less than 50 Thanas. Which indicates that area wise the role and operational coverage of these NGOs are not very significant i.e., 93 percent of these NGOs cater the need of only 10.8 percent of the Thanas. Spatial dimension of programme coverage of the NGOs are therefore still quite low.

As far as direct beneficiaries are concerned, 54 percent of the NGOs

---

[2] Thana is the lowest administrative unit in Bangladesh. There are 460 Thanas in Bangladesh.

cater the needs of less than 30000 potential clients. However this figure is also not the actual programme beneficiaries but is based on the calculation of the population in the catchment areas of the NGOs.

Table 3. Thana Coverage of Health Project NGOs in Bangladesh

Thanas Covered	Number of NGOs	Percentage	Cum Freq.
01 –10	116	71.60%	71.60%
11 –20	18	11.11%	82.72%
21 – 50	16	9.88%	92.59%
51 – 100	5	3.09%	95.68%
101 – 300	3	1.85%	97.53%
Above 300	4	2.47%	100.00%
Total	162	100.00%	0.62%

* Data for 29 NGOs were not available

Table 4. Number of Beneficiary Covered by the Health Project

Number of Beneficiaries	Number of NGOs	Percentage	Cum Freq.
Less than 1000	5	3.13%	3.13%
1000 – 2000	11	6.88%	10.00%
2000 - 5000	23	14.38%	24.38%
5000 - 10000	20	12.50%	36.88%
10000 - 30000	28	17.50%	54.38%
30000 - 50000	16	10.00%	64.38%
50000 - 100000	21	13.13%	77.50%
100000 - 500000	20	12.50%	90.00%
500000 - above	16	10.00%	100.00%
Total	160	100.00%	

* Data for 31 NGOs were not available

On the basis of the tables we may draw the following broad observations:

- In line with the donor priority, the NGOs in health sector emerged significantly during the 1980s. The growth rate of NGOs are marginally higher in the peripheral areas than the major cities.
- Area wise coverage of the NGO operation is still limited to only 10.8 percent of the Thanas of Bangladesh.

ROLE OF NGOS IN HEALTH PROJECTS: CASE-STUDY OF TWO SELECTED PROJECTS

A preference for NGOs over the GOs as an option for delivery of public services is now emerging as a common strategy for donor agencies in Bangladesh. NGOs are identified as an alternative institutional framework to address the problems of local community. Major donors argue that the NGOs have developed an unique understanding of local institutions and of socio-cultural environment and have been able to make valuable contributions to Bangladesh's socio-economic development (World Bank: 1996).

In the following section an attempt has been made to examine two projects run by NGOs to supplement GOB efforts in organisation and management of public health delivery system. These projects are funded by the donor agencies. Both projects are experimental collaborative project between the Government and the NGOs.

The main focus of this review is to highlight the institutional features and the viability of GO-NGO collaborative model in health sector in Bangladesh. To analyse the institutional viability of collaborative model, the study primarily focus on: *how the participating agencies of both GOB and NGOs look in to the project and its viability as collaborative project between government and NGO sector.*

The study choose two projects run by BRAC and CARE in collaboration with Ministry of Health and Family Welfare (MOHFW) as case studies. The Family Planning Facilitation Project (FP-FP) of BRAC and Child Health Initiative for Lasting Development (CHILD) project of CARE have been selected for the case study.[3]

ASSUMPTIONS OF THE PROJECTS

Both of these projects are based on the following assumption:

- NGOs are well organised, planned and action oriented compared to GOB functionaries;
- NGOs have considerable experiences in approaching and mobilising the rural population at large;
- GOB functionaries at the grass root level are weak in project design, implementation, supervision and monitoring;

---

[3] In the study researchers interviewed a total of 75 respondents, taking 25 each from CARE, BRAC and MOHFW field offices involved with those two projects. In addition, several observation visits were made to the project areas. Some discussion sessions were held with the senior officials of CARE, BRAC and MOHFW at the national headquarters in Dhaka.

- GOB functionaries   of the MOHFW lack planning and management skills at the operational level;
- NGOs can supplement the GOB programme operation through transfer of soft technology and management planning and skills;

Accordingly the GOB and the concerned NGOs made a collaboration agreement to design and implement the project with a view to:

- supplement GOB's family planning programme / Child survival services in peripheral areas;
- enhance the quality of care of its services;
- implement innovative means for social mobilisation and communicate supplement service   delivery in areas with gap;
- works towards increased community involvement and sustainability of programme effects and   achievements;
- assist GOB in the implementation of national programmes through replication of experiences a   nd models from BRAC and CARE.

CASE STUDY-I: FP -FP OF BRAC

Bangladesh Rural Advancement Committee (BRAC) is a well established national NGO. It has been working with a view to empower the rural poor and alleviate poverty in Bangladesh. BRAC has already gained a world-wide reputation for its various successful development oriented programmes. International observers have identified BRAC as one of the most effective Bangladeshi NGOs which has challenged development orthodoxy and successfully promoted a new *people- centred* approach for development (Clark 1995).

With the encouragement from the international donor agencies , BRAC has been showing interest to be a partner with the government of Bangladesh in organising and management of health sector projects in the peripheral Bangladesh. One such example is BRAC assistance in GOB's *Expanded Programme on Immunisation (EPI)*. Areas recorded a significantly high rate of immunisation where BRAC was involved in facilitation of the government programme. Success of the collaboration with BRAC further encouraged the GOB to develop new areas of collaboration in health sector.

In the early 1990s, the Government of Bangladesh through the Ministry of Health and Family Planning Welfare, (MOHFW) requested BRAC to assist in implementing the Mother and Child Health and Family Planning (MCH-FP) sector projects in the country. BRAC was specially requested to focus on some of the low performing areas to enhance the contraceptive coverage and develop a strategy leading to sustainability of the MCH-FP achievements. BRAC's Health and Population Division (HPD) therefore initiated the Family Planning Facilitation Programme (FP-FP) to facilitate family planning activities in four low-performing districts i.e. Nilphamari, Sherpur, Hobigonj and Moulvibazar. This programme is being funded by the USAID through Pathfinder International.

The FP-FP programme was initiated in December 1994 to augment the quality of life through improved maternal and child morbidity and reducing mortality. In its first year of operation, the programme was implemented in the eleven-(11) Thanas of Nilphamari and Sherpur districts. From the second year i.e. from December 1995, the project activities were expanded to all the fourteen-(14) Thanas including the three municipalities of Hobigonj and Moulvibazar districts. Presently FP-FP programme is operated in twenty-five Thanas of the four districts. FP-FP programme covers a population of 5.3 million and provides management and training support to the national population programme of the MOHFW.

To begin with, BRAC field level staff undertake a diagnostic survey and collect grass-root level information on health related issues and local needs. The BRAC diagnostic survey identifies the weaknesses of GOB programmes and the causes of low performance. BRAC staff then present the findings of the study in joint meeting of BRAC and the field level MOHFW staff. Based on the findings of the survey and diagnostic study, BRAC's staffs provide technical assistance to the GOB staff at the district level to prepare a comprehensive work plan with a view to enhance the quality of care of its services. In joint working sessions BRAC staff assist the GOB staff to prepare the comprehensive work plan. On the basis of the comprehensive work plan, operational programme plans are designed in close consultation and support from BRAC. BRAC staff assist the MOHFW filed level functionaries to revise and readjust the operational plans. In addition BRAC provides management supports, management information support, training support and also provides facilitation of government services centres (satellite clinics, sterilisation camps and EPI outreach centres). Besides BRAC's staff help mobilising the target group. The field workers of BRAC also make the target group aware of the service facilities through proper counselling.

The implementation of the programme is supervised jointly through field visits by the BRAC and MOHFW field staff. BRAC collects feedback from the clientele through the field level staff. This feedback helps the project team to modify the action plan and develop future work plan.

In summary the FP-FP is a collaboration project to:

- enhance the professional skills of the field staff of MOHFW ;
- to train and develop the managerial capacity for planning and delivery of services;
- to assist and provide technical support to MOHFW field staff to design intervention strategies and monitoring system;
- to co-ordinate the activities at the grass-root level in conjunction with the groups mobilised by BRAC.

CASE STUDY II: CHILD HEALTH INITIATIVE FOR LASTING DEVELOPMENT (CHILD) OF CARE:

CARE International is the world's largest private, non-sectarian non-for-profit relief and development agency[4]. CARE has been functioning in the area now known Bangladesh since 1955. Prior to independence in 1971, CARE was primarily involved in relief activities, school and pre-school feeding and construction of warehouses and low cost housing. CARE has worked closely with GOB and local agencies since 1971 with a view to achieve a sustainable impact on rural poverty.

Brief History of CHILD Project: In October of 1991, GOB took an initiative to improve the overall health status of children and women of reproductive age and GOB requested CARE to assist in this programme. As a result in collaboration with the MOHFW, CARE- Bangladesh has developed the Child Health Initiatives for Lasting Development (CHILD) project in Sylhet district. In the first phase, the CHILD project had been implemented in five of eleven Thanas of Sylhet for a four year period. Based on the lessons-learned from the project, Phase II of CHILD has been launched in September 1995 to cover additional three Thanas of Sylhet district under newly created Sylhet division.

The overall purpose of CHILD- II is :

- to improve the delivery of child survival services through the existing MOHFW system in order;
- to increase access to and use of health services at the community level.
- to strengthen the MOHFW's capacity to deliver high quality, sustainable and integrate outreach services by establishing closer

---

[4] Since 1946 CARE has assisted people in more than seventy-five countries on five continents to improve their quality of life. Currently, CARE operates development assistance and disaster relief programmes in forty Asian, African and Latin American countries. These programmes directly address basic needs of the poorest people through primary health care, agriculture and natural resources and small enterprise development.

linkages between MOHFW field workers, the community and local NGOs.

In order to achieve these project goals CARE do the following activities:

- promote and support a broad community mobilisation and education component through transfer of skills to MOHFW field workers;
- mobilise key community members and use different community women groups of NGOs/GOB and the household owners of outreach sites as community mobiliser;
- provide technical assistance to MOHFW for implementation of child survival services through planning and organising of satellite clinics and outreach centres;
- offer on the job training to the MOHFW service providers;
- assist in maintaining EFI cold chair and the supply of family planning logistics to organise satellite clinics assists MOHFW managers to monitor and analyse the performs, and
- respond to MOHFW priority programmes and to local needs through assists to plan and implement national events such as National Immunisation Day and Maternal and Child Health Fortnight successfully..

A functional analysis of the role of CARE in the project indicate the following areas of its involvement in the project:

a. training for transfer of skill to the MOHFW;
b. maintaining link with community and the MOHFW field functionaries;
c. provide technical assistance for planning, resource mobilisation and organising out-reachprogrammes.

IN BOTH PROJECTS THE ROLE OF THE NGOs ARE CONFINED TO THE FOLLOWING ACTIVITIES

1. Collection of grass-root level data and information for planning and diagnostic assessment;
2. Community mobilisation for programme delivery and effective community participation;
3. Undertake community based awareness training;
4. Assistance in designing an operational plan for the GOB officials at the field levels;
5. Provide management support and training to the field staff of the GOB;
6. Assist in developing and installing a monitoring, evaluation and feedback system;

7. Technical assistance to the professional staff of GOB in planning, decision making, action plan design, and operational plan development;
8. Impart on the job training to the GOB field staff.

Based on the observation visits and structured field level interviews some basic observations have been drawn by the study, which are as follows:

A significant proportion of the field level functionaries of both GOB and NGOs (BRAC and CARE) involved in the collaborative projects noted the importance and necessity of such collaboration projects in the health sector. Almost all respondents from the NGOs noted the importance of such collaborative projects, though few GOB functionaries hold some reservations regarding the strengths of such collaboration with the NGOs. They noted that the NGOs are over stretching their functional boundaries and trying to marginalise the efforts of the GOB at the grass-root level.

GOB functionaries and the NGO officials however noted the following strengths of such collaboration projects:

- It has developed a unique grass root level network for programme implementation;
- The approach of GO-NGO collaboration has introduced an innovative programme management style;
- It has created a condition of mutual learning and transfer of knowledge and technology both ways;
- It has ensured quick response to local need;
- The system has helped in mobilising local opinion and ideas;
- It has reduced the extent of red- tapism;
- Ensured a greater degree of peoples' participation;
- Introduced an efficient planning system;
- Enhanced the over all efficiency in identification of target groups / clientele needs and problems;
- Created a professional environment and capacity for monitoring and evaluation.
- Also enhanced local accountability in programme delivery system;

Some weaknesses of the collaboration model are also identified. These include:

- It has developed inter-organisational conflict;
- It has created a scenario of donor dependency on the part of the GOB as well as NGOs;
- In the name of dual supervision and monitoring it has created a situation of mutual mistrust;

- It is not cost effective and has created a dualism in programme operations;
- Because of strong donor connections, NGOs tend to dominate the implementation and decision making process;
- Because of personality clashes between the GOB and NGO programme officials, decisions in many cases are delayed and has caused the rate of project implementation;
- The system of joint / dual supervision and monitoring have created some confusion in terms of unity and line of command ;and
- Because of design errors in supervision, support and decision making process, the model has created a situation of cold war between the GOB and NGO staff. A strong "we" and "they" feeling is persistent in the project. This feeling of mistrust has caused the performance of the project significantly.

In general NGO staff hold a positive approach towards the project. They seem to be sincere and serious in the implementation process of the project. Because of a strict monitoring system for both operation management and staff control & accountability, the overall performance of the NGO staff are satisfactory and visible. Moreover the NGO staff seem to have developed a harmonious working relationship with the clientele.

GOB staffs, on the other hand, appears to be passive and reluctant about the project. GOB field staff are found to be very much self-guarding and conservative as regards to the relationship with their NGO counter parts. A significant portion of the GOB staff interviewed by the study group seem to suffer from some kind of "superiority complex" as being more educated, trained and being a tenured government staff[5]. The GOB staff noted that NGO staff tend to over rule their decisions made "undue interference" in daily operations in the name of dual supervision. They also attempt to "steal away" the achievements and credits of the GOB field level functionaries. Some GOB functionaries even questioned the "technical competence" of their NGO counter-parts.

However the attitude of the GOB officials vary at the upper level (mostly in the District and Directorate level). During our interviews with GOB officials at the upper level, we found them to be quite positive about the project. They appreciated the contributions made by NGO counterparts and noted that this type of project in actuality has contributed a base for

---

[5] In a traditional society like Bangladesh, a job in government service is always considered to be a matter of social prestige and recognition.

mutual benefit and learning to cater the need for challenging task of development management in Bangladesh.

PROBLEMS-IDENTIFIED IN COLLABORATIVE PROGRAMMES

Based on our preliminary observations we may draw following conclusions:

- There appears to be some built-in design errors in the GO-NGO collaboration project model;
- Faulty design has caused problems of dual authority, supervision and decision making;
- The GOB officials at the grass root level have not been properly briefed or oriented about the spirit, content and operational modalities of the project;
- The GOB officials at the grass root level never had any structured monitoring system to appraise their role and function. With the introduction of joint monitoring and supervision system, on the job training by an external agency, most MOHFW officials feel threatened and insecured and thus resisted the project.
- The project as a matter of fact failed to take into account the dominant bureaucratic culture of the GOB functionaries at the grass root level.
- The NGO officials maintain a very good relations with the clientele. They undertake extensive field visits and follow up trips. NGO officials also enjoy a very good logistics support like transport, office and other support services. On the other hand their GOB counterparts do not have enough logistics support. Thus at the operational level, the GOB staff feel "frustrated" and are "demoralized" and consequently develop a passive resistance to the project as such and NGO counter parts in particular.

On the basis of the observations and field information, the study recommends the following:

- to review the basic premise and working assumptions of the collaboration project;
- to examine the project operational manual and address the built-in structural limitations of the ·project;
- to organise an elaborate reorientation and de-briefing sessions for both GOB and NGO functionaries at the grass root level;
- to bring more transparencies and openness as regards to the project goals, objectives, policies and strategies - which would

develop a better understanding between the two partners.

CONCLUSION

The overall findings of the study indicate that the project has indeed added a new management style in the delivery of health services. It has significantly enhanced planning capabilities of the receiving partner i.e. GOB health functionaries at the grass root level. The project has also updated the level of working knowledge and understanding of local problems by of the GOB officials. More strikingly it is noted that due to the impact of the project, the field level functionaries of the GOB have become more open to the local people. The project has been successful in developing better communication with local government and the community and thus is able to develop a platform for popular participation in health care system and management.

Given the rich experiences of the NGOs in Bangladesh, it is neither possible nor desirable to ignore the role of NGOs in development management specially in a critical sector like health and family planning. A healthy GO-NGO relationship can only be conceived where both parties share common objectives and strategies. With a view to utilise the potentials of both the sectors, a genuine partnership could be developed between NGOs and the GOs on the basis of mutual respect, acceptance of autonomy, independence and pluralism of opinions and positions. Both the partners should recognise the fact that collaboration is a long term affair and it should be developed on mutual trust and respect which would ensure utilising the potentials of both the sector and bringing mutual benefits.

REFERENCES

ADAB (1994): *Fact Sheet on NGO Activities.* Dhaka : Association of Development Agencies in Bangladesh (ADAB)

Aminuzzaman, S, & Nunn, E. (1994): *Institutional Framework of Poverty Alleviation in Bangladesh.* SIFAD TA Project, UNDP, Dhaka.

Aminuzzaman, S. (1993): "Development Management And the Role of NGOs In Bangladesh" *Administrative Change,* Vol.19, No.2.

Asian Development Bank (ADB) (1992): *Cooperation With NGOs in Agriculture and Rural Development in Bangladesh.* Dhaka: ADB

Asian Development Bank (ADB) (1993): *An Assessment of the Role and Impact of NGOs in Bangladesh.* Asian Development Bank

Bhattacharya, Debapria & Ahmed, Salehuddin (1995): *GO-NGO collaboration in Human Development Initiatives in Bangladesh.* BIDS Research report No. 139, Dhaka: BIDS

Clark, J. (1991): *Democratizing Development : The Role of Voluntary Organizations*. Connecticut: Kumirian Press,

Clark, John (1995): "The State Popular participation 'and The voluntary sector, " *World Development*, Vol. 13, No.4.

Farrington, J. & Bebbington, A. (1993): *Reluctant Partners: Non-governmental Organizations. The State and Sustainable Agricultural Development*. Non-Governmental Organizations Series. London: ODI

Huda, Khawja Shamsul (1987): "The Development of NGOs in Bangladesh", *ADAB NEWS*,. No. May-June.

Korten, David C. (1991): The Role of Non-governmental Organization in Development: Changing patterns and Perspectives. In: Paul, S. & Israel, A. (eds.): *Non-Governmental Organizations and the World Bank: Cooperation For Development*. Washington, D. C.: World Bank

Paul, S. (1991): NGOs and The World Bank: An Overview. In: Paul, S. & Israel, A. (eds.): *Non-Governmental Organizations and the World Bank: Cooperation For Development*. Washington, D. C.: World Bank

Shelly, M. R. (1992): *NGO Movement in Bangladesh*. Working Paper, Dhaka :Centre for Development Research.

World Bank (1996): *Pursuing Common Goals: Strengthening Relations Between Government And Development NGOs*. Dhaka: World Bank Resident Mission

17. The shifting missions of NGOs: BRAC in Bangladesh

A.K.M. Saifullah

Introduction

Bangladesh has been experiencing almost three decades of massive NGO activities with the poverty alleviation agenda on the forefront. However, there has not been any spectacular advancement in the status of the poor, the ill-fated 50% of the population. Nevertheless, Bangladeshi NGOs have become world-famous and role models for many people and institutions developing and donor countries alike. Among them is the Bangladesh Rural Advancement Committee (BRAC). With its more than 50.000 paid staff it is perhaps the largest NGO in the world.

During the past thirty years the NGOs in Bangladesh have gone though a remarkable transformation. For the poor, the NGOs first appeared as relief giving organizations. Later they came across some organized groups working with dedication for the rehabilitation of the war ravaged people of the country. Afterwards NGOs are appeared as the catalysts for development, the poor being provided with financial services to change their fate themselves. In this road the NGOs concentrated more on women as these segments of population in Bangladesh were really in jeopardy. Nowadays NGOs can be found in some business, which is hardly in harmony with their earlier missions. When we talk about NGO activities we must consider the premise of NGO activities and what the poor are really getting

This paper focuses on the Bangladesh NGO scenario with special emphasis on BRAC as the pioneer of NGO activities in large scale. The central issues include: a) the shifts in missions i.e. commercialization of NGOs in Bangladesh and BRAC in particular, b) credit operation and empowerment of the poor i.e. women and c) in quest for institutional sustainability

NGOs in Bangladesh: The New Empire

Bangladesh is a fertile ground for NGOs. Contemplating the free reign of foreign NGOs, the local experts also come forward to form NGOs with the aim to alleviate poverty, as poverty still is, according to the WHO (1995), 'the world's deadliest disease'. The contemporary literature on development often cites NGO activities as traditions in this part of the world. In the current estimate Bangladeshi NGOs cover 78 per cent of the villages in Bangladesh and about twenty four million people (approximately one-fifth of the population) benefit from their activities. And these NGOs in Bangladesh spend $500 million (Tk.2350,00,00,000)[1] funds approved by the foreign donors for implementing different projects (Haq, 1997). In another conservative estimate NGOs in Bangladesh spent $12 billion (Tk. 600 billion) in last twenty years (Inqilab, 7 October, 1998).

NGOs in Bangladesh are therefore another significant sector (may it be called as third sector) for development other than the public sector and the private business sector. On the way to the endless journey of the NGOs towards eradication of poverty, the number of entourage is gradually increasing, with no real change in the poverty situation in Bangladesh. The NGOs in Bangladesh are sometimes called Private Voluntary Development Organization (PVDOs) (Holloway, 1998) in line with the US fashion. No doubt at the outset there were people involved voluntarily in the NGOs in Bangladesh. However, with the passage of time they have consolidated themselves into something differently and their practices have been gradually changing. People now find the NGOs doing business in the name of helping the poor in alleviating their poverty.

The history of massive NGO intervention in development in Bangladesh is as old as three decades. From the early age to today the people have experienced different dimensions in the NGOs. In fact the colonial church-based organizations made the NGO concept popular in Bangladesh with a humanitarian face. At that time the Missionaries were engaged in serving the distressed people with food, medicines etc. But during the natural calamities (1970) and man made calamities like the war of independence (1971) the people received different types of services from the NGOs. These activities include relief and rehabilitation assistance to the misfortunate people. Initially after the independence in 1972 Bangladesh Rehabilitation Assistance Committee (BRAC) had come into being to salvage the distressed people of the country. BRAC was in fact was a positive response to the needs by some young, educated and patriotic people.

The next shift of NGO activities was in the mid seventies when NGOs perceived that relief and rehabilitation are not enough for the poor people in Bangladesh. So they devote themselves in the aim of developing

---

[1] US $ = Tk. 47 (author's calculation)

the living standard of the rural poor in Bangladesh what popularly known as 'poverty alleviation program'. The main focus of such program on the part of NGOs was poverty alleviation through raising the consciousness and provides them with money they lack to sustain their life. NGOs do believe that they are helping individuals and communities to become self-reliant with the ultimate objective of ending the long standing exploitative relationship that dominate rural life in Bangladesh. In 1973 BRAC changed the philosophy of their mission and rename the organization as Bangladesh Rural Advancement Committee (BRAC) keeping the initials intact (Chowdhury & Alam, 1997). It started to think providing their assistance collectively to the community rather than individually, and began calling the activity Community Development Program.

In late 1970's with all other programs, NGOs gave more importance on awareness rising and income generating programs. For these programs to be successful NGOs followed a more concentrated ways to reach the real needy people to serve. This is called target group approach. BRAC accepted target group approach as their policy in 1976. At the same time microcredit as piloted by the Grameen Bank became popular among NGOs. So a principal occupation for NGO sector in Bangladesh became collecting members for receiving credit from them. The credit venture of NGOs is very profitable one as they charge a higher interest rate than commercial banks.

In the nineties a new dimension has been added in the NGO activities in Bangladesh. They are not happy with the profits from credit activity. Sustainability has become talk of this decade. NGOs in Bangladesh responded well to the concept of sustainability. They face the quest for sustainability by engaging in business. They manifest the impression that to make the people self-reliant they have to become self-reliant first. And eventually keeping this impression in mind NGOs have started establishing commercial enterprises. Also here BRAC played the pioneering role in establishing printing press and shops of selling rural crafts called ARONG. ARONG has its shops in home and abroad. Nowadays BRAC has more than fifteen commercial ventures (see Annex 1).

From the above discussion it is clear that voluntarism is gradually disappearing from the NGO sector in Bangladesh and NGOs are now more interested in doing business. This is really the concern of the time. NGOs are now the reality in Bangladesh. In many areas of Bangladesh society NGOs have contributed in a way or other. But the new trend of NGOs in getting involved in business is a dangerous signal to the poverty alleviation efforts of the nation. By nature business tends to make profit. And the businessman is not concerned about the welfare of the customer. By shifting the focus to profit making exercises the NGOs are approaching the poor people of Bangladesh with new intentions that can prove to be harmful to the disadvantaged majority.

BRAC'S CREDIT PROGRAM AND EMPOWERMENT OF THE POOR

The main program of BRAC is the Rural Development Program (RDP) where a credit activity is the primary one. According to BRAC, the main thrust of RDP is to develop a viable village organization[2] (VO) for the landless at the grassroots, make them critically aware of the environment in which they live, and to initiate measures of changes to improve the conditions of their life and work. These organizations are the main vehicle of BRAC intervention in rural development. A VO gets matured through a long process, such as, organizing the landless into groups, development of village organizations, imparting functional education tom the group members, holding group meetings, encouraging savings and group fund formation, and training. In this way institutionalization has occurred which BRAC deems very important.

BRAC's Savings[3] and *Credit* (see Annex 2 for the features of BRAC credit program) program is to help create a financial base for the group members through savings mobilization and credit so that they can carry out different income generating activities. BRAC's current credit program, developed over the years through many trial and error, is now one of the largest in the world with more than 38 million US dollars in members' savings and 469 US dollars as loan disbursed (BRAC, 1997).

BRAC's credit program is familiar one in Bangladesh. Following the philosophy given by Professor Md. Yunus that 'the poor of Bangladesh are bankable' and inspired by the success of Grameen Bank, NGOs in Bangladesh have taken the mission to alleviate poverty through microcredit. It is basically a neo-classical economic approach. Credit raises the family income. The income is allocated to satisfy the different needs of the household, there by increasing the welfare of the family. A general income increase pushes the rural economy and leads to overall economic growth

---

[2] Organization means Village Organization (VO) developed by the Program Organizers (POs) of BRAC, helping mobilization of target man and women in a given locality. A VO comprises of approximately 40 members with eight to ten small groups of five or less. Members must have no or less than five decimals of land. The age bar is between 18-54 years.

[3] There are two ways a VO member saves money; she saves a minimum of Tk. 2per week on the average or she deposits 5% of the loan she takes from BRAC into her savings account.

(ASA, 1997). BRAC practices the same features in credit program what was initially known as Grameen Bank product. The very features of this credit program are i) small size of loan, ii) guarantee by a group instead of a collateral, and iii) repay through weekly installments.

Bangladesh has proven to be fertile land for NGO microcredit activities. There is a broad consensus that in order to get out of this poverty crisis it is required to engage the poor in non-agricultural professions and income. And for such engagement of these groups of people, institutional credit is essential. Credit is seen as a fundamental right of the poor beside other basic human rights. Credit is considered far better than any kind of relief. It is believed that credit makes the poor responsible, self-interested, active, self employed and production oriented. So the logic is that credit should not be considered as a hand-out and it must involve a cost. The NGOs in Bangladesh therefore engaged in distributing credit with high enough interest that it covers the costs or even generates profit.

Though credit is regarded an ideal means to alleviate poverty in Bangladesh especially by the NGO sector, there are also other views. Dr. Nizamuddin Al-Hossainy, the Additional Director, Department of Women's Affairs, Government of Bangladesh thinks: "For the poorest, micro-credit for self employment is not going to be their first need, or indeed what they need at all- a secure means of saving, or consumption loans to see them over all illness for example, might be much more important" (Observer, Feb. 7, 1997).

The concept of collateral free credit with collective responsibility to the group is now popular all over the world. The program has its objective in mind that to save the poor from the moneylenders who charge high interest on their loan given to the poor people in rural Bangladesh. BRAC is one of the four "big players"[4] in Bangladesh which focus on "Credit to the poor", with about 2.23 million members and an annual credit disbursement of Tk. 6.9 billion in 1997 exceeding the previously set targets (BRAC, 1997).

In some development literature the NGOs capacity in reaching poor is highlighted (Smillie & Helmich, 1993; Farrington & Bebbington, 1993). But in fact the NGOs in Bangladesh, including the big players and BRAC as well, have very limited capacity to reach the poorest of the poor, the most vulnerable group in the society. In the "International Workshop on Poverty and Finance in Bangladesh: Reviewing the Two Decades of Experience" held in Dhaka, it was concluded that NGOs "have made a significant contribution to poverty alleviation but have had a much more limited

---

[4] The four big players are Grameen Bank, BRAC, Proshika and ASA are standing according to the amount of loan disbursement. For details see- ASA, 1997

impact on poverty removal". The workshop summery also notes that 'the high expectations held of Micro Credit Institutions (MCIs) has at times led to the false impression that they can solve the problem of poverty' (Khan & Amin, 1997; for the case of BRAC see also Hashemi, 1999).

When writing in the 25 year progress report of BRAC Ian Smillie (1997) found that it is synonymous with efficiency, effectiveness and all the best meanings that can be attached to the word 'development'. He also added the new targeting policy of BRAC, was aimed primarily at the very poorest. But researchers are not on the way of such claims. Among Bangladeshi researchers Hashemi (1992) found that large NGOs in Bangladesh fail to reach the poorest in their efforts to achieve rapid expansion in geographical coverage—the drive for "breadth" rather than "depth". Dr Hossain Zillur Rahman and Dr. Mahbub Hossain of BIDS on their study on poverty pointed out that, in spite of the almost exclusive status of credit within the menu of poverty alleviation programs, access to credit is still limited to only a quarter of rural household, indicating still significant scope for expansion of such programs. Credit access is relatively higher among the moderate poor and this group received 31% of total loan disbursed (Grameen Trust, 1996, p. 10).

If we consider the poverty, based on the extent of receiving credit it is revealed that compared to the similar organization BRAC's performance poor. From the research of Khandaker & Chowdhury (1996) it is found that among BRDB (a government run program), Grameen Bank and BRAC, the record of the last mentioned organization is worst. Unlike with the other organizations, the members of the BRAC credit programs were becoming more impoverished the longer they participated in the activity (see, Table 1).

Table 1: Poverty based on the extent of receiving Credit *(Percentage of participants; Month based)*

Organization	Moderate Poverty			Absolute Poverty		
	<12 m	12-24 m	24+ m	<12 m	12-24 m	24+ m
BRDB	83	--	67	63	33	6
Grameen Bank	80	88	59	20	35	8
BRAC	63	86	70	12	14	14

Source: Khandaker & Chowdhury, 1996, p. 263

While analyzing the influence of credit on poverty Asaduzzaman (1997) mentioned that in terms of participation in credit program and its influence on poverty, the track record of BRAC is worst among similar organizations. Thus independent researchers have not empirically proved the worldwide notion of NGOs supremacy in managing the poverty alleviation programs. And BRAC is an ideal example to supplement the above statement.

THE PREFERENCE FOR WOMEN CLIENTS

BRAC likes to manifest itself as an advocate of social change. For bringing effective social change the first priority is to end all kind of discrimination in the society be it sexual, racial or any other kind. For effective social change in Bangladesh, empowerment of women is the first thing to do. No doubt, the poorest women are disadvantaged especially because they do not have access to information and resource. So they are lagging behind in the process of development. BRAC would like to involve these women and enhance their participation in the development process with the view that ultimately the participation will bring them out of the cycle of poverty. It states that there is a strong desire to increase women's well being and engages them in activities that would empower them socially and economically. BRAC deems empowerment is rooted in sustainable gain for women through measures like awareness building, credit and savings, and profitable income generation. Therefore, women are the best chosen clienteles in credit program of BRAC.

In credit program BRAC's Program Organizers (POs) are trained in such a way that they think 'credit' is the one and only way to the empowerment for the poor rural women. But researchers doubt about the mission of NGOs who are working towards empowerment of women. As Rutherford finds not for empowerment but some other practical reasons are almost wholly responsible for the move to an exclusively female clientele. These practical reasons are (for details see Rutherford, 1995):

- women are at home during the day and can be reached during normal working hours;
- they appear more likely to repay loans on time;
- they are more pliable and patient than men and so less likely to make awkward demands on the scheme managers;
- they can be serviced by women staffs who are cheaper to employ than men;
- Bangladeshi women are usually simple and trustworthy;
- they have no numerical knowledge to rightly calculate the installments and interest rates.

By 1997 BRAC has given credit to 2.23 million borrowers of which 98 per cent are women. (BRAC, 1997). In business there is less inclination to invest money into activities where there is high risk. To make its investment risk free BRAC has chosen women as clients. The recent World Bank study also reveals that *"defying conventional wisdom, who make up about 90 percent of the total borrowers, have proven to be excellent credit risks, with a rate of default that is less than one third that of man"* (Khandaker, 1998).

The practice of microredit is far from ideal. Many loans given to women are captured by men. They take it and use it but it is the women who have to meet the repayments, sometimes denying themselves food to pay the loan. Tension can build between wives and husbands when the men do not pay up. Examples abound where women have taken loans and ended up worse of then ever.

This way NGOs like BRAC use women empowerment programs for business interest. In lieu of empowering women BRAC looks primarily for prospective loanees. At the same time BRAC is conspicuously silent about the severe violence against women, an issue that should be a major concern for any group dealing with women's empowerment. Of the violence most common are rape, domestic violence, dowry related cases and acid burn attacks. BRAC has through their publication and media been critical only about *fatwas*[5] against women but hardly mentioned the other issues.

BRAC now and then tries to sell the idea that it has succeeded in bringing out the female to participate in the economic activities. It is said that these women had broken the situation of keeping them tied with *purdah*. In fact researchers see that it is not NGOs credential but the pressures of survival (endangered by economic and demographic shifts arising from the differentiation of the peasantry) have left little option to the majority of households amongst the landless and assetless classes other than to permit their women to take part in market-based income-earning activities (Adnan, 1989).

BRAC IN QUEST OF INSTITUTIONAL SUSTAINABILITY

During the past decade donor agencies have been putting increasing pressure for the NGOs to become less dependent on the foreign aid. The problem of high unit costs of NGOs and their tendency build own permanent institutions with funds meant for temporary 'project'' interventions have been highlighted. This quest for 'sustainability' has lead NGOs to increase their other sources of income, such as interest from credit programs and profits from commercial ventures. BRAC with its more than fifteen enterprises is a case in point.

---

[5] The literary meaning of Fatwa is the verdict based on Shriah, the Islamic code of conduct and ethics. Some times the little learned so-called religious leaders mislead the people by giving distorted explanation of Shariah.

"To reach and benefit the poor more meaningfully Microfinance Institutions (MFIs) must work towards institutional financial self-sufficiency (IFS)"— this was the main theme of Microcredit Summit Campaign 1997. This institutional self-sufficiency will make the MFIs competent to operate at a level of profitability, and eventually allows the organizations in reducing dependence on donor money. The result will be development of a sustainable strategy of service delivery to the poor (for details see, Gibbson & Meehan, 1999). The only measure in this end as believed by Gibbson and Meehan that these organizations have to be commercially motivated and strategy will be go after profit. It was only in 1997 when financial self-sufficiency became a major issue internationally, but BRAC in Bangladesh had taken this policy long before the Summit.

Gibbson and Meehan's version of IFS clearly states that there is no doubt that the poorest should pay full cost for their financial services but they should not be asked to bear the burden of NGO credit program's incompetent management and inefficient operations. So the case is that the poor have to bear the cost of the service they receive. And if an credit providing NGO shows lower management capacity the poor may face a real danger. The following table will show how vulnerable the poor are while they accept the services of NGOs. The study on comparative operational cost per group member enrolled in various NGO and government credit programs by Alam (1988) showed that the operational cost of NGO sponsored programs is very high. This study is some older, the situation remain same to date with slight improvement.

Table 2: Cost of Operation of NGOs and GOs

Name of the Organization	Cost per Member (Tk.)
Grameen Bank	383.56
BRAC	936.88
RDRS	1962.41
Proshika-MUK	308.45
Swanirvar	22.42
BRDB	173.24

Source: Alam, 1988, p. 88

The operating cost of BRAC programs per member in 1988 was Tk. 936.88. The poor group members are paying this cost as they are paying higher interest than other sectors. It is sure that by paying this amount unknowingly, the helpless poor are becoming more vulnerable.

Another study (though some older but significant in this case) conducted by Canadian International Development Agency showed the aspects of sustainability of NGO programs (Table 3). The study presented the perception of group members about the future of their programs. The group members were of the view that their income would decline if NGO withdraws from the area. Nobody answered affirmative that his/her income would be further improved. In case of BRAC programs 62% of the respondents opined that their income would decline if it withdraws from the working area. And only 38% said that the income would remain unchanged.

Table 3: Sustainability of NGO programs*

Name of the Organization	No. of Respondents	If NGO withdraws from the area what would ˪ ᴜᴇ income status		
		Would be further improved	Would remain unchanged*	Would decline
ASA	49	--	2 (4)	47 (96)
BRAC	39	--	15 (38)	24 (62)
PROSHIKA-MUK	45	--	20 (44)	25 (56)
RDRS	20	--	20 (44)	6 (30)
GRAMEEN BANK	25	--	7 (28)	18 (72)

*(According to the Perception of group members,) * Number in the parentheses indicates percentage.
Source: CIDA , 1985, p.49*

The group members view were also found justified when it was revealed that "nowhere has BRAC phased out, which proves that before a group becomes self-reliant, much has to happen. The existing group have not expanded on their own, nor have they succeeded in changing their economic condition more than marginally" (Chowdhury, 1996, p. 109). And in 1999 Syed Hashemi proved the same when he writes, ... there is no indications of successful NGO withdrawal from any area (Hashemi, 1999). After almost three decades of operation the situation remains the same. From this situation one may conclude that, NGOs don't really want to change the life of the poor significantly, or they have limitation in their capacity to do the same. The other answer may be that any significant change in the rural life will make the presence of NGOs difficult. The reason is that if a poor man/woman become self-reliant s/he will never come back to receive NGO credit. NGOs are not so foolish to do loose their prospective clients by making them self-reliant.

NGOs often say they are supplementing government initiatives to alleviate poverty and that the programs will be phased out after gaining certain level of upliftment of the poor. Such program will then be initiated in other new areas. But very few instances, if any, are found where an NGO leaves an area after attaining some level of success. Rather they are building permanent structures of their own. For BRAC it is very much the case: "BRAC policy makers have developed from the days when they spurred institution building, leaving it to the government authorities, now they are aiming at building permanent structures" (Chowdhury, 1996).

The recent Bangladesh Bank survey titled "A Study on the Flow of Credit in Rural Activities 1998" provided some messages of concern. In this study it was found NGO credit programs are in jeopardy, though the number credit organizations are increasing. NGOs don't officially admit the situation but contemplating among themselves. This is why the concept of financial self-sufficiency has arrived in the credit scenario. In this compelling situation BRAC is has chosen to go for commercial ventures long before other NGOs. A few of the commercial ventures of BRAC are as follows:

Delta-BRAC Housing Finance Company Ltd.: It is the first of its kind in Bangladesh in private sector. It is created to finance people willing to build or purchase houses (apartments) in Dhaka. The company is a joint venture of Delta Life Insurance Company Limited and BRAC, Green Delta Insurance Company Limited from Bangladesh, Housing Development Finance Corporation (HDFC) India and International Finance Corporation (IFC), one of the arms of the World Bank. From where the share of BRAC's capital has come in this venture? Perhaps, these are the money from the rural Bangladeshi poor that save with BRAC as a counter part fund for their loans, they received from BRAC or this money has come to make BRAC self-sufficient. Does donor give money to join a multi-national using their money? But the fact is that BRAC has made link to international finance capital and becoming business tycoons in Bangladesh. It is also an indication that NGOs are really the product of the New International Economic Order.

BRAC Printers is one of the biggest and technologically most developed printing house in Bangladesh. BRAC Printers as enjoying a status of not-for-profit organization, import papers, inks and other machinery's getting tax exemptions. Thus BRAC Printers is offering more competitive price than other printing firms and getting more contracts. BRAC Printers is enjoying NGO status and getting tax exemptions but doing commercial business with the raw materials that were imported in the name of voluntary activities.

BRAC is selling computers (**BRAC Computers**), providing Internet and e-mail services (**BRAC BD Mail Network**) and recently also established an institution named **BRAC Information Technology Institute** (BITI) for developing technical manpower. In this way by purchasing computers, using e-mail and Internet services and taught by high paid tuition fee the son of the poor will become empowered and poverty will no more be a curse for the Bangladeshis.

BRAC Seed and Feed Marketing Project has also been established to sale hybrid rice and vegetable seeds to the farmers. Through this organization the beneficiaries of BRAC credit program are being suggested to purchase these in market prices. They are heading into monopolistic tendency in the name of free market sale.

Nowadays one can see very attractive advertisement of a new Hotel in Dhaka i.e. **Hotel BRAC Centre Inn** in short Hotel BRAC Inn in the Bangladesh dailies and weeklies. This latest version of BRAC business has been established an international standard hotel at the BRAC head office building taking four floors of its twenty-two storied BRAC Centre.

CONCLUDING REMARKS

The above analysis shows that what NGOs have been doing, all in the name of the poor and to provide better services to the poor. In spite all their concerted efforts little has been changed to the life of the poor. Still 52% of the total population living under the poverty line, only 45% of them have access to health service and 34% have sanitation facilities (Haq, 1997). While everything has been laid to the poorest, these segments of the society are getting very little form NGOs. For example, BRAC is not giving credit to the poorest of the poor. Several studies proved this statement true (see Khandker, 1999; Montgomery, 1995; Montgomery and others, 1996). Its prospective clients are the well of households with up to a minimal standard of financial stability and who are able to take risk on investing in small business. Richard Montgomery called this credit as "promotional credit" that promotes business. Montgomery form his vast experience in South Asia and in particular in rural Bangladesh, further argued that 'in South Asia there are millions of poorer household who need "protectional credit" – loans to dig themselves out of ill-health or other emergencies, or to tide over lapses in their income (Montgomery, 1995 cited in Rutherford, 1995).

The poorest are excluded from BRAC's on other grounds as the interest rate is very high and essentially that micro credit institution should be profitable and cost effective, in order to reach ever larger number of clients. Larger number of clients means more profit. And this profit will be further invested in some big projects (Delta BRAC Housing Company Ltd.) as it developed. Where is the end of this trend?

And when BRAC fails to reach to the poorest how can it justify the high rate of interest (usually far more than market but lower than traditional moneylenders) as commercialization of credit has been suggested to reach them. How will then the poor become empowered? Who will enjoy the benefit of institutional self-sufficiency? How far NGOs or in this case BRAC has to work in the grassroots level if there found no instances of withdrawal form any where? Perhaps only time will say what BRAC will become through establishing giant commercial enterprises?

REFERENCES:

ADAB (1994), *Fact Sheet on NGO Activities,* Dhaka : ADAB

Aminuzzaman, S, and   E. Nunn,(1994), *Institutional Framework of Poverty Alleviation in Bangladesh,* SIFAD TA Project, UNDP, Dhaka.

Aminuzzaman, S: 1993: "Development Management And the Role of NGOs In Bangladesh" *Administrative Change,* Vol.19, No.2.

Asian Development Bank (ADB) (1992), *Cooperation With NGOs in Agriculture and Rural Development in Bangladesh ,* ADB Dhaka

Asian Development Bank (ADB), (1993), *An Assessment of the Role and Impact of NGOs in Bangladesh,* Asian Development Bank.

Bhattacharya, Debapria and Salehuddin Ahmed: (1995), *GO-NGO collaboration in Human Development Initiatives in Bangladesh:* BIDS Research report No. 139, Dhaka: BIDS

Clark, J, (1991) *Democratizing Development : The Role of Voluntary Organizations,* Connecticut, Kumirian Press,

Clark, John: (1995), "The State Popular participation 'and The voluntary sector, " *World Development,* Vol. 13, No.4.

Farrington J. and Bebbington A : 1993, *Reluctant Partners : Non-governmental Organizations, The state and Sustainable Agricultural Development,* Non-governmental organizations series, ODI, London.

Huda, Khawja Shamsul, (1987). *"The Development of NGOs in Bangladesh",* *ADAB NEWS,. No. May-June.*

Korten, David C, (1991), "The Role of Non-governmental Organization in Development: Changing patterns and Perspectives" Paul, S and A. Israel (et. al) *Non-governmental Organizations and the World Bank: Cooperation For Development,* Washington, D.C.; World Bank

Paul, S: 1991, "NGOs And The World Bank: An Overview", Paul S and A. Israel (et. al) *Non-governmental Organizations And The World Bank; Cooperation For Development,* Washington, D.C. World Bank.

Shelly, M.R (1992), *NGO Movement in Bangladesh,* Working Paper, Dhaka

:Centre for Development Research.

World Bank (1996), *Pursuing Common Goals: Strengthening Relations Between Government And Development NGOs*, World Bank Resident Mission, Dhaka.

ANNEX: 1 THE LIST OF BRAC'S COMMERCIAL ENTERPRISES:

1) BRAC Housing Ltd
2) ARONG Marketing Outlet
3) BRAC Bank
4) BRAC BD-Mail Network
5) BRAC Cold Storage LTD.
6) BRAC Computers
7) BRAC Dairy (ARONG Milk)
8) BRAC Institute of Information Technology
9) BRAC Printers
10) BRAC Publications
11) BRAC Seed and Feed Marketing Project
12) BRAC Steel Mills
13) BRAC Textiles
14) BRAC Transport
15) BRAC University
16) Delta-BRAC Housing Finance Company Ltd.

Source: BRAC Library, Newspapers and other printed Documents.

ANNEX 2 FEATURES OF BRAC CREDIT PROGRAM

Features	Description
Membership criteria	Maximum landing holding of .5 acre of land. At least one household member must work for wages (since 1992 one member allowed per household)
Group features	30-40 members from village organizations. Village organizations are divided into solidarity groups of 5-7 members. Separate groups for men and women. Each women group has a counterpart men group. Weekly meetings of solidarity groups.
Savings mobilization	Tk. 2 per week. 4 percent of each loan (nonrefundable) goes to group fund. 1 percent of each loan used for group insurance.
Credit delivery mechanism	No collateral but group liability. 50 week installment of loan. Interest at the end of loan cycle. 20 percent interest for production loans. Maximum loan Tk. 1000.
Social development	Training duration 3-6 months. Review of code of conduct (see Appendix.6) at village organization meetings. Substantial skill-based training.

Source: Khandker, 1999, p. 24

Box 2

MICRO-CREDIT AND EMPOWERMENT OF POOR WOMEN IN BANGLADESH

Salma Akhter

Micro-credit and income generating activities for rural women are central elements in the development initiatives of NGOs in Bangladesh. Since the mid-1980s special credit institutions in Bangladesh have dramatically increased the credit available to poor rural women. The 1980s brought increasing pressures from promoters of gender-sensitive development policy in domestic development community of Bangladesh as well as among its foreign aid donors for the inclusion of women in rural credit and income generating activities.

To find out about the relationship between women-focused activities of an NGO to increase women's contribution to household income and the resultant impact on their status within household and in the community a study of one of the Bangladesh's largest NGO, Proshika, was conducted by the author. The primary data collection was based on PRA in Manikgonj, Madaripur, Barisal districts where Proshika credit programmes have presence. Furthermore, a household survey was done which included information on household demographic composition, holding of lands, cattle before and after being member of NGO credit-group. Some personal case studies were done as well.

Both rural and urban Proshika members feel that they have control in decision making inside household and as well as at community level. Being in administrative decision making; getting access to social power by being involved in different committees; having greater mobility; talking to outsiders; opposing and lessening social injustice, like violence against women, dowry, polygamy, divorce, crime; self-assertion and social prestige are very common indicators of empowerment within the Proshika members. Proshika members mentioned that because of their consciousness, unity and group action they have reduced number of incidences of social inequality and social injustice that they count as a success and as an indication of empowerment.

Regarding economic empowerment, majority of women have income generating activities and identified their extra income as necessary as well source for affording a little luxury that raised their status within the family and community level also. Proshika members mentioned about having physical violence, verbal abuse from husbands and in-laws, specially mother-in-law before becoming Proshika members which they feel reduced up to 90 percent after their involvement with Proshika group. Most of them mentioned of having peaceful and honourable lives because of their contribution to alleviate poverty in their families as their group solidarity encourages and supports them in need and provides access to social institutions that help them to be empowerment socially.

Regarding control over credit-money, it is more apparent in the slum women as they are investing their money themselves and repaying loan from their own earnings. In rural sites in most cases, women usually invest credit money in leasing lands, invest in husband's or son's shops except in some cases of buying livestock or doing homestead gardening. In most cases husbands or sons control money and they repay the money so the credit recipient women are not aware of the profit and exact amount of return from this money. Control over money or enjoying dominating role in family did not appear as a strong indicator in the agenda of poor women. Most of them do not consider verbal abuse of husbands as a repressing or abusing behaviour. To a group member, 'if I do not do any wrong, he is nice to me, if I can't take care of him when he is back home after hard work, it is natural that he will be rude to me'.

It is evident from the study that providing training with credit is more powerful than just providing credit to alleviate poverty of poor women as women become more aware of utilising credit money after receiving training which provide knowledge and opportunity for income generation activities. Most women members receiving credit without training usually take loan to support male members of family. Form the study it appears that the training and credit facilities don't reach equally to all Proshika members. Proshika members involved in social committees are receiving training and credits several times comparing to other members. None the less, these women are conscious of their rights and status and perceive that they are empowered after being involved in the group based micro-credit programmes of Proshika.

A good number of women in these areas who are hard-core poor regretted that most members don't include poorest for group formation as other members are afraid that they may not be able to repay loans, so these women are being deprived of social empowerment as well. Most Proshika members view the insufficient gap between receiving loan and the 1st instalment of repayment are difficult for the credit recipients as most people cannot invest their money and get return by that time for repayment. They also perceive the interest rate as high for poor recipients. Credit recipient women opine that these two factors are hindering the desired rate of poverty alleviation. Lack of constant/stable source of income and natural disasters are major problems for economic empowerment and sustainability of the poor women. Proshika's Thana cordination's savings fund aims to work as future insurance and sustainability of poor.

There are few cases of women members who are leaving Proshika group as they find the provision of attending weekly meetings inconvenient and have to be penalised for default members. On the other hand, it is evident from the study that hard core poor are left out and are deprived of NGOs credit programmes and training facilities as they can't get into a group because of their inability to repay loan immediately as they are landless, mostly widows or abandoned women, old. A good number of women in Madaripur and Manikgonj study areas showed their interest to be in groups not only just for receiving credit or training but also for the psychological, social and economic support from group members.

Ms. Salma Akhter is Assistant Professor of Sociology at the University of Dhaka, Bangladesh.

Box 3

THIRD SECTOR IN BHUTAN

Dhurba Rizal

In view of its natural and self imposed isolation that existed till 1960, pattern of economic activity in Bhutan has been simple. Planned development commenced in 1961. Since then, Bhutan has implemented seven five-year economic development plans, ushering limited progress in different sector of economy to uplift the living and quality of life of Bhutanese people. With the advent of planned development in 1961, certain changes in economy were inevitable.

Bhutan is mostly dependent upon the development partners for financing the development plans. Government is the sole formulator, implementers, organisers and evaluator of development activities with limited participation of INGOs, NGOs and local community organisations. Just like any other developing nations of Asia, Africa or Latin America, the notion of aid or assistance has been associated with religious activities. Bhutan is a state founded as the theocratic framework by re-incarnating Lama in 16th century. Thus, people donated land and resources to monasteries and temples. Serving the poor, disabled and helpless people was widely practised in ancient day Bhutan.

The seed of an INGOs was first transplanted into Bhutanese soil in 1950s, when Leprosy Mission of Norway and HELVETAS of Switzerland came to Bhutan at the initiative of Government. Save the Children Fund of USA make its inroad sometime in 1960s. In 1980s, the government set up National Youth Associates of Bhutan (NYAB). At the same time, bilateral and multilateral donors like JICA, DANIDA, CIDA came to Bhutan as developmental partners. In 1990s, the government set up the Royal Society for Protection of Nature (RSPN) to protect the environment and wildlife. To boost the people to people contact, few association emerged in foreign soil at the initiate of royal family.

The setting up of National Women's Association of Bhutan (NWAB) on 9th April 1981 to ensure the participation of women in development was a concrete step in paving the way for non-governmental organisations.. It functioned as non-ministerial government department from 1985 to 1991. It undertakes schemes for improvement of the socio-economic conditions of women throughout Bhutan by identifying the constraints that women face and suggest appropriate solutions. Many of the activities of the NWAB are carried out by voluntary women's association members both in the capital and in the districts while head quarter's staff act as a link between the Royal Government Ministries and the Dzongkhag's (Districts). It has a total of about 450 voluntary members.

However, any Government initiated organisation may not succeed with its mission as it is totally controlled by the royal family and mostly used to mobilised for their own vested interest. Moreover, it has no mass based institutions. The participation of people is limited by lack of institutional linkages, funds, managerial capacity and suitability of policies and programs to local people. It is a government sponsored and economically supported organisations and it may soon dissipate merely as an organisation, churning out policies in sharp contrast to the autonomy and independence with which they are supposed to deliver the objectives in mind. It has hardly raise any voice, when more than hundred thousand people from south and east was forcefully evicted, tortured, raped and assaulted by government and security forces. If this is the trend, it may just wither away as just another government agency rather than nurturing as a true voluntary agency alive to the needs of segment it tend to serve and participate in developmental efforts.

The exodus of people since 1990 to escape the atrocities and prosecution of the regime provided a fertile breeding ground for the emergence of NGOs in exile. As of now, there are around forty nine NGOs operating to advocate the cause of the suffering refugees and raising the voice against the atrocities of regime. Few political organisations were also formed to pressurise the regime to demoralise the state and guarantee the basic fundamental rights of people. Most of the NGOs are involved in advocacy but NGOs like BRAVE (Bhutanese Refugee Aiding the Victim of Violence), Refugee Women Forum are involved in skill development and income generations. The BRAVE and Refugee Women were established in exile to provide humanitarian assistance to the victim of violence in Bhutan. It was a structured response initiated by a group of like mined individuals who or whose family members, relative or friends have had become the victims of violence at the hands of security forces in Bhutan after the 1990's pro-democracy and human right movement. Their major objectives in exile was to rehabilitate the victim of violence in confidence building, economic activities in order to enable to recoup their original vigour and strength to make a normal living in the refugee camps.

Most of the NGOs in exile work with relief agencies such as UNHCR, SCF, LWS, WFP, Red Cross. On the positive side, they are acquiring and developing advocacy skill, leadership qualities, empowerment of weaker sections of society, but on the other hand they are not cost effective. The resources channelled to many of the NGOs, without clear cut objectives are not properly utilised for desired cause. People involved in NGOs are manipulating funding sources and alienate themselves from the community, making their objectives more alien and unsustainable. NGOs in exile are first generations NGOs, mostly engaged in relief and welfare strategies. Many NGOs in exile are in the hands of opportunistic forces which are hiding behind the so called "Good NGOs" facade.

The scope of NGOs involvement in Bhutan is vast, but existing authoritarian rule of regime pre-empt the emergence of reformist NGOs. Moreover, the political turmoil has been the biggest obstacles to the proliferation of indigenous NGOs. Whatever NGOs has been mushroomed in exile, it has not been recognised by government. Existing NGOs either created at the initiative of govt. or in exile are weak and lack capabilities to design, organise and manage development program.

Mr. Dhurba Rizal is currently associated with the Central Department of Public Administration, Tribhuvan University.

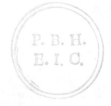